Current Issues in Treatment of Osteochondral Defects

Editor

MARK S. MYERSON

FOOT AND ANKLE CLINICS

www.foot.theclinics.com

Consulting Editor
MARK S. MYERSON

March 2013 • Volume 18 • Number 1

ELSEVIER

1600 John F. Kennedy Boulevard • Suite 1800 • Philadelphia, Pennsylvania, 19103-2899

http://www.foot.theclinics.com

FOOT AND ANKLE CLINICS Volume 18, Number 1
March 2013 ISSN 1083-7515, ISBN-13: 978-1-4557-7088-5

Editor: David Parsons

Foot and Ankle Clinics (ISSN 1083-7515) is published quarterly by Elsevier, Inc., 360 Park Avenue South, New York, NY 10010-1710. Months of issue are March, June, September, and December. Periodicals postage paid at New York, NY, and additional mailing offices. Subscription price per year is $299.00 (US individuals), $401.00 (US institutions), $148.00 (US students), $341.00 (Canadian individuals), $473.00 (Canadian institutions), $204.00 (Canadian students), $439.00 (foreign individuals), $473.00 (foreign institutions), and $204.00 (foreign students). To receive student/resident rate, orders must be accompanied by name of affiliated institution, date of term, and the *signature* of program/residency coordinator on institution letterhead. Orders will be billed at individual rate until proof of status is received. Foreign air speed delivery is included in all *Clinics* subscription prices. All prices are subject to change without notice. **POSTMASTER:** Send address changes to *Foot and Ankle Clinics*, Elsevier Health Sciences Division, Subscription Customer Service, 3251 Riverport Lane, Maryland Heights, MO 63043. **Customer Service: 1-800-654-2452 (US and Canada). From outside of the United States and Canada, call 314-447-8871. Fax: 314-447-8029. E-mail: JournalsCustomerService-usa@ elsevier.com (for print support); JournalsOnlineSupport-usa@elsevier.com (for online support).**

Reprints. For copies of 100 or more, of articles in this publication, please contact the Commercial Reprints Department, Elsevier Inc., 360 Park Avenue South, New York, NY 10010-1710. Tel.: 212-633-3812; Fax: 212-462-1935; E-mail: reprints@elsevier.com.

Printed and bound by CPI Group (UK) Ltd, Croydon, CR0 4YY
Transferred to Digital Printing, 2013

Contributors

CONSULTING EDITOR

MARK S. MYERSON, MD
Director, The Institute for Foot and Ankle Reconstruction, Mercy Medical Center, Baltimore, Maryland

EDITOR

MARK S. MYERSON, MD
Director, The Institute for Foot and Ankle Reconstruction, Mercy Medical Center, Baltimore, Maryland

AUTHORS

ALEXEJ BARG, MD
Orthopaedic Department, University Hospital of Basel, Basel, Switzerland

GREGORY C. BERLET, MD
Orthopedic Foot and Ankle Center, Westerville, Ohio

JAMES D.F. CALDER, TD, MD, FRCS(Tr&Orth), FFSEM(UK)
Chelsea and Westminster Hospital; Fortius Clinic, London, United Kingdom

REBECCA CERRATO, MD
Foot and Ankle Fellowship Program, The Institute for Foot and Ankle Reconstruction, Mercy Medical Center, Baltimore, Maryland

WOO JIN CHOI, MD
Department of Orthopaedic Surgery, Yonsei University College of Medicine, Seoul, South Korea

DANIEL J. CUTTICA, DO
The Orthopaedic Foot & Ankle Center of Washington DC, Falls Church, Virginia

VINCENZO DENARO, MD
Chelsea and Westminster Hospital; Fortius Clinic, London, United Kingdom

PREMJIT PETE S. DEOL, DO
Panorama Orthopedics and Spine Center, Golden, Colorado

NORMAN ESPINOSA, MD
Department of Orthopaedics, University of Zurich, Balgrist, Zurich, Switzerland

PAUL HARRISON, BSc
Head of OsCell, Trauma and Orthopaedic Department, Robert Jones and Agnes Hunt Orthopaedic and District Hospital, NHS Trust, Oswestry, Shropshire, United Kingdom

JOON JO, MD
Department of Orthopaedic Surgery, Yonsei University College of Medicine, Seoul, South Korea

BEN JOHNSON, MBBS, BSc
Orthopaedic Specialist Registrar, Trauma and Orthopaedic Department, Robert Jones and Agnes Hunt Orthopaedic and District Hospital, NHS Trust, Oswestry, Shropshire, United Kingdom

JACQUES JONCK, FCS Orth(SA)
The Institute for Foot and Ankle Reconstruction, Mercy Medical Center, Baltimore, Maryland

ANISH R. KADAKIA, MD
Department of Orthopedic Surgery, Feinberg School of Medicine, Northwestern University, Chicago, Illinois

PATRICK LAING, MBBS
Consultant Orthopaedic Surgeon, Trauma and Orthopaedic Department, Robert Jones and Agnes Hunt Orthopaedic and District Hospital, NHS Trust, Oswestry, Shropshire, United Kingdom

JIN WOO LEE, MD, PhD
Department of Orthopaedic Surgery, Yonsei University College of Medicine, Seoul, South Korea

CAROLINE LEVER, MBBS
Orthopaedic Specialist Registrar, Trauma and Orthopaedic Department, Robert Jones and Agnes Hunt Orthopaedic and District Hospital, NHS Trust, Oswestry, Shropshire, United Kingdom

UMILE GIUSEPPE LONGO, MD, MS
Department of Orthopaedic and Trauma Surgery, Campus Bio-Medico University, Trigoria, Rome, Italy

MATTIA LOPPINI, MD
Department of Orthopaedic and Trauma Surgery, Campus Bio-Medico University, Trigoria, Rome, Italy

NICOLA MAFFULLI, MD, MS, PhD, FRCS(Orth)
Centre for Sports and Exercise Medicine, Barts and The London School of Medicine and Dentistry, Mile End Hospital, London, United Kingdom

NILESH MAKWANA, MBBS, FRCS(Orth)
Consultant Orthopaedic Surgeon, Trauma and Orthopaedic Department, Robert Jones and Agnes Hunt Orthopaedic and District Hospital, NHS Trust, Oswestry, Shropshire, United Kingdom

BERT R. MANDELBAUM, MD, DHL(Hon)
Santa Monica Orthopaedic and Sports Medicine Group, Santa Monica, California

HELEN MCCARTHY, BSc
Researcher, Trauma and Orthopaedic Department, Robert Jones and Agnes Hunt Orthopaedic and District Hospital, NHS Trust, Oswestry, Shropshire, United Kingdom

GRAHAM A. MCCOLLUM, FCS Orth(SA), MMED(UCT)
The Institute for Foot and Ankle Reconstruction, Mercy Medical Center, Baltimore, Maryland; Chelsea and Westminster Hospital; Fortius Clinic, London, United Kingdom; Department of Orthopaedic Surgery, The University of Cape Town, Groote Schuur Hospital Observatory, Cape Town, South Africa

AMY MORGAN, MBChB, MRCS
Department of Trauma and Orthopaedic Surgery, University Hospital of Wales, Cardiff, United Kingdom

MARK S. MYERSON, MD
Director, The Institute for Foot and Ankle Reconstruction, Mercy Medical Center, Baltimore, Maryland

ANTHONY PERERA, MBChB, FRCS (Orth)
Department of Trauma and Orthopaedic Surgery, University Hospital of Wales, Cardiff, United Kingdom

JAMES RICHARDSON, PhD
Professor of Orthopaedics, Trauma and Orthopaedic Department, Robert Jones and Agnes Hunt Orthopaedic and District Hospital, NHS Trust, Oswestry, Shropshire, United Kingdom

SALLY ROBERTS, PhD
Director of Spinal Research, Trauma and Orthopaedic Department, Robert Jones and Agnes Hunt Orthopaedic and District Hospital, NHS Trust, Oswestry, Shropshire, United Kingdom

GIOVANNI ROMEO, MD
Department of Orthopaedic and Trauma Surgery, Campus Bio-Medico University, Trigoria, Rome, Italy

WILLIAM BRET SMITH, DO, MS
Moore Orthopedics, Lexington, South Carolina

RACHEL TRICHE, MD
Santa Monica Orthopaedic and Sports Medicine Group, Santa Monica, California

VICTOR VALDERRABANO, MD, PhD
Orthopaedic Department, University Hospital of Basel, Basel, Switzerland

C. NIEK VAN DIJK, MD, PhD
Department of Orthopaedic Surgery, Academic Medical Center, University of Amsterdam, Amsterdam, The Netherlands

NAVIN VERGHESE, MB.BS (Lond), FRCS (Orth)
Department of Trauma and Orthopaedic Surgery, University Hospital of Wales, Cardiff, United Kingdom

MARTIN WIEWIORSKI, MD
Orthopaedic Department, University Hospital of Basel, Basel, Switzerland; Center for Advanced Orthopedic Studies, Beth Israel Deaconess Medical Center, Harvard Medical School, Boston, Massachusetts

Contents

This article reviews the basics of articular cartilage biology, which provide a necessary foundation for understanding the evolving field of articular cartilage injury and repair. The currently popular treatment options for osteochondral injury (microfracture, osteochondral autograft transfer system, osteochondral allograft, autologous chondrocyte implantation, and the use of scaffolds with autologous chondrocyte implantation) document the significant advances made in this area in the past 2 decades. Integration of newly available information and technology derived from advances in molecular biology and tissue engineering holds even greater promise for continued advances in optimal management of this challenging problem.

In this article, our research on osteochondral lesions of the talus (OLTs) is summarized, the orthopedic literature is reviewed, and the direction of future research and treatment trends are discussed. Our research has explored the role of lesion size, significance of marrow edema, relationship of patient age, importance of lesion containment, and role of a stable cartilage lesion cap in the prognosis and outcomes of these lesions. We have identified smaller sized lesions, younger patients and contained lesions as independent predictors of success for the operative treatment of OLTs. Our data should facilitate the development of a more comprehensive treatment algorithm to more accurately predict success in operative management of these lesions.

Acute bone bruises of the talus after ankle injury need to be managed differently from osteochondral defects. Bone bruises have a benign course, but there may be persistent edema. A bone bruise should not delay rehabilitation unless symptoms persist or significant edema is close to the subchondral plate. Osteochondral defects have a less predictable prognosis, and rehabilitation should aim at promoting healing of the subchondral

(OATS) an excellent option for recurrent, deep, or moderate defects. For defects with a large diameter, large cystic component, or heavily involving the shoulder of the talus, an allograft provides an excellent option. This article focuses on the efficacy and determination of the most appropriate graft reconstruction: allograft reconstruction or OATS.

Osteochondral lesions of the talus are generally benign, and many heal or are not symptomatic. A subset of these defects progress to large cystic lesions, which have a less favorable prognosis. The treatment options are joint preservation or sacrifice. Joint salvage entails marrow stimulation techniques or hyaline cartilage replacement with allograft or autograft. When lesions reach greater than 3 cm^2 or Raikin class IV or become uncontained on the shoulders of the talus, autografting techniques become more challenging. Osteochondral allografting may be a better surgical option, often achievable without a malleolar osteotomy for exposure.

Cell cultured techniques have gained interest and popularity in osteochondral defects because, unlike bone marrow stimulation methods, where fibrocartilage fills the defect, they allow for the regeneration of "hyaline-like cartilage" with better stiffness, resilience, and wear characteristics. Osteochondral defects in the ankle are a rare but challenging problem to treat in young active patients. If left alone, they can cause pain and reduced function and risk progressive degenerative changes in the joint. Clinical results of cell cultured and scaffold technology in the ankle, although still limited by small studies and midterm follow-up, are certainly encouraging.

Recurrent ankle sprains and other trauma as well as ankle malalignment can lead to chronic osteochondral lesions of the talus. Conservative treatment frequently fails. Several operative treatment techniques exist; however, the choice of the right procedure is difficult. This article presents a new surgical technique suitable for treatment osteochondral lesions that combines bone plasty and a collagen matrix.

Preface
Osteochondral Lesions of the Talus

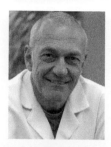

Mark S. Myerson, MD
Editor

I recall when the only treatment for an osteochondral lesion of the talus was arthroscopic debridement. Try to imagine what our treatment alternatives will therefore be in another 30 years! I believe that our understanding of these lesions is still evolving and, while we really cannot predict trends in treatment, I suspect that these will be directed biologically rather than mechanically. Although the outcomes of many of our current surgical procedures are exciting, I remain skeptical about any new trendy procedure since the literature is replete with successes as well as failures of these initiatives. I frequently hear about new techniques from colleagues and friends but find these to be overly optimistic. Many surgeons adopt a new procedure (and I am guilty of this myself), only to move on a year or 2 later to the next and newest treatment alternative. And whether it is a new type of cartilage resurfacing or alternative method of grafting, I do not know of any treatment that has a really predictable outcome. The rate of success has hovered around 80% for decades despite multiple treatment alternatives, but the only procedure to have stood the test of time is debridement and microfracture. This is, of course, as we well know, not a satisfactory biologic treatment, and yet many, indeed the majority, of the patients do quite well. How willingly do you, the surgeon, embrace new ideas and technologies? We have many alternatives for treating the large cystic lesion where the results of debridement and microfracture are not satisfactory and this issue will certainly highlight all of the current and future options for treatment.

Mark S. Myerson, MD
The Institute for Foot and Ankle Reconstruction
Mercy Medical Center
301 St Paul Place
Baltimore, MD 21202, USA

E-mail address:
Mark4feet@aol.com

Foot Ankle Clin N Am 18 (2013) xi
http://dx.doi.org/10.1016/j.fcl.2012.12.011
1083-7515/13/$ – see front matter © 2013 Published by Elsevier Inc.

foot.theclinics.com

Erratum

An error was made in the December 2012 issue of *Foot and Ankle Clinics* (Volume 17, number 4) on page 555. Two of the authors of "Total Ankle Replacement for Rheumatoid Arthritis of the Ankle" were listed incorrectly. The correct author names are Sean Y.C. Ng and Xavier Crevoisier.

Foot Ankle Clin N Am 18 (2013) xiii
http://dx.doi.org/10.1016/j.fcl.2013.01.001

Overview of Cartilage Biology and New Trends in Cartilage Stimulation

Rachel Triche, MD*, Bert R. Mandelbaum, MD

KEYWORDS

- Osteochondral • Articular cartilage • Injury • Lesion • Stimulation • Repair
- Treatment • Management

KEY POINTS

- Understanding the unique biology of articular cartilage is necessary for improving outcomes using current methods and for devising improved methods.
- Most current methods result in creation of fibrocartilage or hyaline-like repair tissue, which is less durable than native articular cartilage.
- New, single-stage surgical methods using implanted chondrocytes or pluripotent cells may improve outcomes.
- Tissue engineering, scaffolds, and use of growth factors may all help yield grafts composed of hyaline cartilage that mimics native articular cartilage.

BIOLOGY OF ARTICULAR CARTILAGE

Articular cartilage is a highly specialized tissue type with unique characteristics that are functionally important and have significant implications for treatment options. Articular cartilage is avascular and hypocellular and is not innervated. It is composed primarily of water and extracellular matrix. Chondrocytes are the only cell type present and make up a mere 5% of the total weight.[1] There are no mesenchymal stem cells or pluripotent progenitor cells within articular cartilage. This unique composition affords important mechanical properties that allow cartilage to function effectively under the loads transmitted across joints. Mature cartilage is thus by definition a poor source of regenerative tissue, resulting in a limited capacity for healing.

Components

Articular cartilage is composed of chondrocytes in an extracellular matrix (ECM) of collagen, proteoglycans, and water. The ECM accounts for 95% of the cartilage

Disclosures: R.T: None. B.R.M: Paid consultant for Zimmer.
Santa Monica Orthopaedic and Sports Medicine Group, 2020 Santa Monica Boulevard, Suite 400, Santa Monica, CA 90404, USA
* Corresponding author.
E-mail address: rtriche@smog-ortho.net

Foot Ankle Clin N Am 18 (2013) 1–12
http://dx.doi.org/10.1016/j.fcl.2012.12.001
1083-7515/13/$ – see front matter © 2013 Elsevier Inc. All rights reserved.

volume and is secreted and maintained by chondrocytes. Type II collagen is the predominant collagen, with type IX and type XI collagen the most prevalent minor collagen types present. Collagen types V, VI, X, XII, and XIV are also present although in limited amounts. Aggrecan is the largest and most abundant proteoglycan. Aggrecan is a highly glycosylated protein that contains 2 types of glycosaminoglycans, chondrotin sulfate and keratin sulfate. Multiple aggrecan molecules bind to hyaluronic acid to form large aggregated proteoglycans that carry a negative charge. This attracts cations, thereby increasing the osmolality, which in turn draws water into the ECM. Other proteoglycans found in articular cartilage include decorin, biglycan, and fibromodulin that all interact with collagen in different capacities to stabilize the ECM.

Chondrocytes are derived from mesenchymal stem cells. They have a low turnover rate and are influenced by growth factors, cytokines, mechanical loads, and piezoelectric forces as well as the surrounding matrix composition. They are also subject to local paracrine effects. Lacking a vascular supply, cell nutrients are delivered by diffusion from the synovial fluid. A complex interaction regulates the balance between synthesis and breakdown of the ECM components by the chondrocytes that is only recently being elucidated. Although the process is intricate, better understanding will likely provide another means of potentially improving the healing potential of cartilage.

Structure

The macrostructure is divided into 4 zones—superficial or tangential, middle/transitional, deep/radial, and calcified (**Fig. 1**). The shape and orientation of the chondrocytes and associated ECM varies in each zone in accordance with the different mechanical loads and stresses. The superficial zone is 10% to 20% of the cartilage thickness. The collagen in this zone is oriented parallel to the articular surface and the chondrocytes are flattened and more dense than in other zones. In the middle zone, 40% to 60% of the thickness, the collagen is more randomly oriented as are the chondrocytes, which are more spherical. The collagen in the deep zone is in bundles that are perpendicular to the underlying calcified cartilage and the chondrocytes are larger and in vertical columns. The calcified zone includes the tidemark that separates the calcified cartilage from the subchondral bone and is integral for the adhesion of cartilage to bone.

Healing potential, as discussed previously, is limited, usually resulting in fibrocartilage formation rather than hyaline cartilage. Fibrocartilage has inferior biomechanical

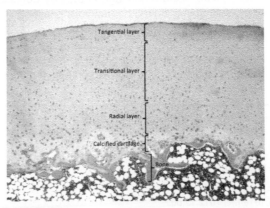

Fig. 1. Zones of articular cartilage.

properties to hyaline cartilage, which leads to degeneration over time and the development of arthritis. Thus, the goal of surgical intervention is to improve and optimize the repair tissue either through indirect means, such as microfracture, to provide access to pluripotent cells with enhanced healing potential, or through direct means, such as chondrocyte implantation or osteochondral grafting.

CURRENT TREATMENTS

Historically the most common treatment of articular cartilage damage was débridement, with the goal of minimizing symptoms. This may alleviate pain for a period of time but does not alter the natural history of the problem. In contrast, newer treatment options aim to have a positive impact on the area of damaged cartilage by providing access to progenitor cells that promote healing of the defect with a cartilage-like material or transplanting cells, either differentiated chondrocytes or pluripotent cells, that can regenerate cartilage.

Current treatment options can be divided into 3 categories: (1) marrow stimulation or reparative techniques, (2) cartilage replacement with osteochondral implantation, and (3) cell-based regenerative therapy.

Marrow Stimulation/Reparative

Marrow stimulation through microfracture is intended to introduce pluripotent cells to the articular cartilage defect by penetrating the subchondral plate and, thereby, eliminating the existing barrier to these cells with healing potential. The blood clot that forms includes mesenchymal stem cells that can differentiate into chondrocytes and produce a cartilage-like repair tissue. The technique has been well described, including the importance of the spacing of the perforations and removal of the calcified cartilage layer to optimize the repair tissue.[2–4] Second-look arthroscopy and biopsy have demonstrated that these lesions heal with fibrocartilage rather than hyaline cartilage.[5] Microfracture has been shown to have good results, particularly in younger patients with smaller lesions in the knee, although recent data in the ankle suggest that while increased size is, age is not an independent predictor of poor outcomes.[6–8] Second-look arthroscopy at 12 months in the talus demonstrated incomplete healing in 40% although the majority had good clinical outcomes as measured by American Orthopaedic Foot and Ankle Society (AOFAS) scores (90% AOFAS scores >80).[5] Midterm MRI and clinical follow-up showed maintenance of the clinical results but evidence of incomplete integration and fissuring in 60% and 100% of cases, respectively.[9] It has also been shown that the positive results tend to decline with time, likely related to the differences in mechanical properties between hyaline cartilage and fibrocartilage repair tissue.[10–14] Microfracture is a widely used technique that is a single-stage procedure with minimal morbidity. The primary disadvantage is the limited durability of the repair tissue, which is fibrocartilage, not hyaline cartilage.

Osteochondral Implantation/Cartilage Replacement

Osteochondral implantation, either allograft or autograft tissue, offers the advantage of a structural replacement at the defect site, including chondrocytes that can produce type II collagen for improved repair tissue composition and underlying subchondral bone (**Fig. 2**). Clinical and MRI data for osteochondral autograft in the talus at an average of 7 years' follow-up show that the osteochondral autograft transfer system provides significant improvement with respect to AOFAS, Tegner, and *visual analog scale* (VAS) scores.[15] Midterm data in 130 patients at an average of 5 years after osteochondral transplantation of the talus demonstrated good results in returning to

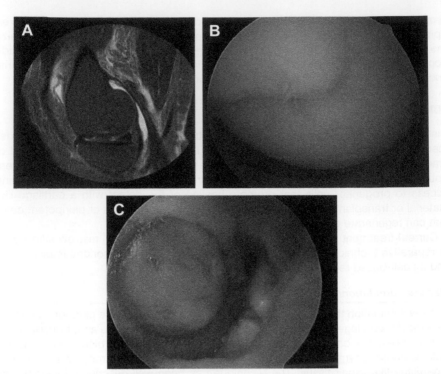

Fig. 2. Osteochondral allograft. (*A*) Preoperative MRI demonstrating full-thickness defect of the medial femoral condyle. (*B*) Arthroscopic image of the full thickness defect measuring 18 mm × 18 mm. (*C*) Final image after osteochondral allograft placed, press fit, and fixed with bioabsorbable pins.

recreational sports, although a shift away from higher-impact activities was noted.[16] The key limitations of the autograft technique are lesion size and donor site morbidity. This has led to the use of fresh osteochondral allograft, which helps overcome those limitations. A recent study of allograft in the talus demonstrated reasonable outcomes at an average follow-up of 37 months, although 4 of 38 grafts failed and 10 of 38 patients rated their results as fair or poor. MRI results were obtained in 15 of the 38 patients and showed maintenance of congruity with limited subsidence and reasonable stability of the grafts.[17] Another recent study of 16 cases demonstrated that 10 of 16 had good outcomes but only 4 of 16 were symptom-free and 5 of 16 were considered failures, with 2 of 16 requiring reoperation.[18] Potential downfalls of both autograft and allograft transplantation procedures include graft subsidence, lack of peripheral integration, and peripheral chondrocyte death. Longer-term follow-up data in the knee suggest that although perhaps these techniques have better durability than microfracture, there is still a time-dependent decrease in survival results with osteochondral transplantation techniques.[19] There is, thus, an unmet need for more durable intervention methods.

Cell-Based Regenerative Therapy

Cell-based transplants have garnered increasing attention as a potential means of addressing the long-term poor outcomes observed with prior methods. The first report of successful transplantation of autologous chondrocytes in the knee was by Brittberg and colleagues in 1994.[20] Chondrocytes are harvested from a non–weight-bearing portion of the knee and expanded in vitro before reimplantation in a second procedure into the defect underneath a periosteal flap. Promising results have been demonstrated with autologous chondrocyte implantation (ACI) in the knee, based on symptom relief, function, and return to sports, including high-impact activities.[21–24] A second-generation ACI technique uses a collagen membrane rather than a periosteal flap to cover the transplanted chondrocytes. This eliminates the need for harvest of the periosteal flap and eliminates periosteal overgrowth, which is a known complication with the first-generation ACI technique, requiring débridement in 18% to 33% of patients.[25,26] Unfortunately, with the second-generation method, chondrocyte hypertrophy can occur and expansion results in dedifferentiation of the chondrocytes such that the cells begin producing type I rather than type II collagen.[27] With any of these transplantation techniques, an osteotomy is frequently necessary to allow adequate access to the lesion, which carries with it additional potential complications, including nonunion and the increased morbidity and restrictions required to allow for healing of this additional procedure.

Thus, there are several commonly used current treatment options with promising results that also present areas for potential improvement. None, however, has yet yielded the desired result, namely, a hyaline cartilage articular surface comparable to the original articular cartilage.

NEW TRENDS IN CARTILAGE STIMULATION

New and emerging treatment options focus on a multimodal approach to optimizing the repair tissue in the treatment of articular cartilage defects. Increased knowledge of the biology of chondrocyte differentiation and signaling provides one means to ultimately enhance repair techniques. Many of the methods emerging from this enhanced understanding focus on the ECM. Tissue engineering advances, including improved scaffolds and matrices for chondrocyte or pluripotent stem implantation, are another area of regenerative enhancement.

An important aspect of these advances is to allow a move toward single-stage procedures that are arthroscopic or minimally open, thereby decreasing the morbidity associated with 2-stage procedures that also potentially require malleolar osteotomy.

Enhanced Microfracture

Clot stability is an important factor in microfracture. Recent investigations in microfracture technique have focused on improving the adhesion of the clot formed through the use of a polysaccharide polymer, chitosan-glycerol phosphate, which has been shown to improve hyaline cartilage repair in animal models.[28–30] Other research has led to the development of injectable biodegradable hydrogels that also improve stability of the repair clot after microfracture.[31] In an animal model, platelet-rich plasma used in conjunction with microfracture has been shown to improve cartilage repair compared with microfracture alone, though this still did not produce hyaline cartilage.[32] Bone marrow aspirate concentrate has also been studied in conjunction with microfracture in animal models and shown to improve cartilage healing both macroscopically and histologically.[33,34]

Growth Factors

Another area of potential improvement in microfracture technique would be to better guide the growth of the repair tissue in an attempt to produce more hyaline cartilage in the defect. Growth factors play an essential role in the differentiation of pluripotent stem cells. Although these pathways are complex, improved understanding of their mediators and which growth factors are important provide information used to help optimize the environment and encourage hyaline cartilage repair. Transforming growth factor β, bone morphogenic proteins 2 and 7, and insulinlike growth factor 1 are all known to play a role in articular cartilage development and maintenance of the differentiated state.[35-39] Additional studies are required to better understand how these growth factors can be used to direct the repair tissue.

Characterized Chondrocyte Implantation

One current area of concern is the change in chondrocytes once expanded in vitro before reimplantation. Dedifferentiation of the chondrocytes in culture results in loss of predominantly type II collagen repair tissue and the generation of more fibrocartilage composed of type I collagen–based repair tissue instead.[27] Although ACI has shown good results in the talus, identification of molecular markers known to represent a subset of chondrocytes that have been associated with hyaline cartilage formation provides a means to selectively expand type II collagen–producing chondrocytes in this subpopulation.[40] Implantation of these expanded, characterized chondrocytes compared with microfracture in a randomized study has been shown to result in better repair tissue at 12 months,[27] but direct comparison to unselected ACI chondroctye implantation has not yet been reported in the literature.

Scaffold-Associated Implantation

Tissue-engineered cartilage scaffolds seeded with chondrocytes or pluripotent stem cells represent a highly promising option for treatment of cartilage defects. Such scaffolds are likely to support long-term commitment to type II hyaline cartilage synthesis by chondrocytes as opposed to the fibrocartilage that is otherwise observed. This is a reflection of the tissue-specific commitment of a chondrocyte that is a function not only of the cellular commitment but also the environment in which it resides. A scaffold that supports hyaline cartilage differentiation thus is a potentially improved source of transplant material. There are several potential benefits to therapies of this type, including decreased invasiveness of the procedure, which can in certain applications be accomplished in a single surgical procedure rather than requiring 2 operations, and the mechanical properties of these scaffolds may better match the properties of native articular cartilage.[41]

Positive clinical outcomes have been shown in the knee and ankle using both type I/III collagen membrane and hyaluronic acid–based scaffolds with implanted chondrocytes both clinically and radiographically.[42-44] The next step in optimizing these techniques is to eliminate the 2-step procedure. A prospective study of talar osteochondral lesions treated in a single stage with bone marrow aspirate concentrate with a collagen/hyaluronic acid scaffold demonstrated significant clinical improvement of AOFAS scores as well as radiographic and histologic evidence of regenerated tissue that was hyaline cartilge in part.[45] In a rabbit model, platelet-rich plasma on a PLGA (poly[lactic-co-glycolic acid]) scaffold compared with the scaffold alone was found on macroscopic and histologic examination to improve healing of osteochondral lesions.[46] These represent promising techniques that will continue to be evaluated for efficacy and durability of the repair.

Currently work is under way in animal models of articular cartilage repair using a bilayer 3-D agarose gel chondral layer with underlying osteo layer where allogeneic chondrocytes are implanted. This is modeled to match the defect using 3-D data obtained from CT or MRI imaging. Culture with dynamic loading in a bioreactor generates an osteochondral construct that can be implanted to create a functional 3-D implant. Results in the animal model have been positive.[47] This represents an exciting new treatment option that may be effective in humans as well.

Single-Stage Chondrocyte Implantation (Cartilage Autograft Implantation System and DeNovo NT Micronized Cartilage)

The interest in moving toward single-stage procedures that produce hyaline cartilage has led to the development of 2 promising procedures—Cartilage Autograft Implantation System (CAIS) (Johnson & Johnson Regeneration Technologies, Depuy Raynham, Massachusetts) and DeNovo NT (Zimmer, Warsaw, Indiana). CAIS uses particulated autologous cartilage obtained in the same arthroscopic procedure that is then implanted on a resorbable scaffold into the defect. Animal models demonstrated good results with hyaline-like repair tissue at 6 months.[48,49] A randomized controlled trial in humans comparing microfracture and CAIS in the knee showed similar results in terms of repair tissue but better IKDC (International Knee Documentation Committee) scores with CAIS.[50] An important factor to consider in translation of this technique to the ankle is the quantity of cartilage that must be harvested, because the availability in the ankle is limited when compared with the knee. DeNovo NT uses allograft juvenile chondrocytes that are provided in their native ECM in 1-mm cubes that are implanted using fibrin glue (**Fig. 3**). Studies in both animal models and early outcomes in human use demonstrate good results again with the formation of hyaline-like cartilage in the defect.[51,52]

An additional experimental technique under investigation uses micronized and lyophilized cartilage prepared from cadaveric tissue implanted into an articular cartilage defect after microfracture. In a study in baboons, complete filling of the defect with hyaline-like cartilage was shown at 9 weeks.[53]

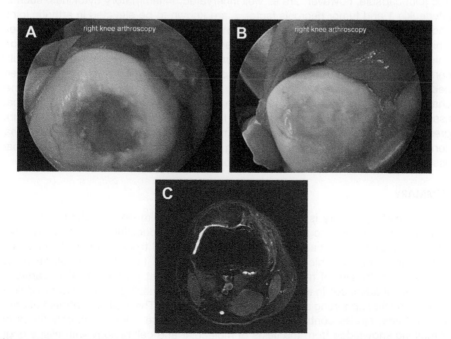

Fig. 3. DeNovo NT. (*A*) Full-thickness articular cartilage defect of the patella. (*B*) After placement of DeNovo NT. (*C*) Follow-up MRI.

Further studies are necessary to determine the indications for use as well as long-term follow-up of these methods, but they represent promising options in cartilage repair with good potential.

Adjunctive Therapies—Pulsed Electromagnetic Field and Gene Therapy

Studies using pulsed electromagnetic fields in a several different animal models have shown increased proteoglycan synthesis and decreased levels of inflammatory cytokines.[54–57] Applications in human studies have shown chondroprotective effects and reduced recovery time after knee arthroscopy.[58] Thus, pulsed electromagnetic field may be a useful adjunct to surgical procedures to maximize recovery while having a positive impact on the repair process.

Gene therapy, using adenoviral transfection of chondrocytes or pluripotent cells, represents an additional adjunctive therapy that may prove powerful in optimizing the treatment of articular cartilage defects. Studies on mesenchymal stem cells transfected with either bone morphogenic protein-2 or bone morphogenic protein-7 and sonic hedgehog have shown improved hyaline cartilage repair tissue.[59,60] Using the expanding knowledge base regarding important growth factors in chondrocyte differentiation and articular cartilage metabolism in the setting of gene therapy presents an additional means to enhance cartilage repair tissue.

DISCUSSION

An interesting issue that is raised when reviewing the treatment options for articular cartilage injuries is the question of pain generation in these lesions and thus how these treatments have an impact on that pain. Articular cartilage is not innervated, so the defect itself is not the source of the pain directly. The subchondral bone, synovium, and joint capsule, however, are all well innervated. Inflammatory cytokines, such as interleukin 1 and tumor necrosis factor α, are known to be elevated in arthritic joints and in turn up-regulate matrix metalloproteinases, aggrecanase and collagenases, which break down the ECM and stimulate nitric oxide prostaglandin E2 production. This inflammatory cascade likely plays an important role in the pain related to articular cartilage injury. This pathway is likely disrupted in 2 ways when undergoing treatment because the synovial fluid is exchanged as a result of the arthroscopy and the biomechanical problem is addressed through the intervention. The breakdown of this repair tissue over time, as is the case with the fibrocartilage generated by microfracture, presumably results in the recurrence of symptoms. If accurate, this possible explanation supports the current aims of improving the biomechanical properties of the repair tissue to generate hyaline cartilage with appropriate subchondral support.

SUMMARY

Articular cartilage injury is a challenging problem. Unlike bone healing, successful cartilage repair requires regeneration of an avascular, hypocellular, multilayered tissue with unique biomechanical properties that are essential to its function. Advances in cellular and molecular biology have provided avenues to guide the cellular repair process with the aim of regenerating chondrocytes that produce hyaline cartilage. Concomitant advances in tissue engineering supply increasingly artful ways to deliver an appropriate supporting structure for the repair tissue. The field of treatment of articular cartilage injuries continues to evolve and the future will undoubtedly focus on combining knowledge from the fields of molecular and cell biology with tissue engineering to optimize the current treatment options and develop novel techniques.

REFERENCES

1. Alford JW, Cole BJ. Cartilage restoration, part 1: basic science, historical perspective, patient evaluation, and treatment options. Am J Sports Med 2005;33(2): 295–306.
2. Mithoefer K, Williams RJ 3rd, Warren RF, et al. Chondral resurfacing of articular cartilage defects in the knee with the microfracture technique. Surgical technique. J Bone Joint Surg Am 2006;88(Suppl 1 Pt 2):294–304.
3. Mithoefer K, Williams RJ 3rd, Warren RF, et al. High-impact athletics after knee articular cartilage repair: a prospective evaluation of the microfracture technique. Am J Sports Med 2006;34(9):1413–8.
4. Frisbie DD, Morisset S, Ho CP, et al. Effects of calcified cartilage on healing of chondral defects treated with microfracture in horses. Am J Sports Med 2006; 34(11):1824–31.
5. Lee KB, Bai LB, Yoon TR, et al. Second-look arthroscopic findings and clinical outcomes after microfracture for osteochondral lesions of the talus. Am J Sports Med 2009;37(Suppl 1):63S–70S.
6. Choi WJ, Park KK, Kim BS, et al. Osteochondral lesion of the talus: is there a critical defect size for poor outcome? Am J Sports Med 2009;37(10):1974–80.
7. Choi WJ, Kim BS, Lee JW. Osteochondral lesion of the talus: could age be an indication for arthroscopic treatment? Am J Sports Med 2012;40(2):419–24.
8. Steadman JR, Miller BS, Karas SG, et al. The microfracture technique in the treatment of full-thickness chondral lesions of the knee in National Football League players. J Knee Surg 2003;16(2):83–6.
9. Becher C, Driessen A, Hess T, et al. Microfracture for chondral defects of the talus: maintenance of early results at midterm follow-up. Knee Surg Sports Traumatol Arthrosc 2010;18(5):656–63.
10. Steinwachs MR, Guggi T, Kreuz PC. Marrow stimulation techniques. Injury 2008; 39(Suppl 1):S26–31.
11. Kessler MW, Ackerman G, Dines JS, et al. Emerging technologies and fourth generation issues in cartilage repair. Sports Med Arthrosc 2008;16(4): 246–54.
12. Gobbi A, Nunag P, Malinowski K. Treatment of full thickness chondral lesions of the knee with microfracture in a group of athletes. Knee Surg Sports Traumatol Arthrosc 2005;13(3):213–21.
13. Robinson DE, Winson IG, Harries WJ, et al. Arthroscopic treatment of osteochondral lesions of the talus. J Bone Joint Surg Br 2003;85(7):989–93.
14. Ferkel RD, Zanotti RM, Komenda GA, et al. Arthroscopic treatment of chronic osteochondral lesions of the talus: long-term results. Am J Sports Med 2008;36(9): 1750–62.
15. Imhoff AB, Paul J, Ottinger B, et al. Osteochondral transplantation of the talus: long-term clinical and magnetic resonance imaging evaluation. Am J Sports Med 2011;39(7):1487–93.
16. Paul J, Sagstetter M, Lämmle L, et al. Sports activity after osteochondral transplantation of the talus. Am J Sports Med 2012;40(4):870–4.
17. El-Rashidy H, Villacis D, Omar I, et al. Fresh osteochondral allograft for the treatment of cartilage defects of the talus: a retrospective review. J Bone Joint Surg Am 2011;93(17):1634–40.
18. Haene R, Qamirani E, Story RA, et al. Intermediate outcomes of fresh talar osteochondral allografts for treatment of large osteochondral lesions of the talus. J Bone Joint Surg Am 2012;94(12):1105–10.

19. Gross AE, Shasha N, Aubin P. Long-term followup of the use of fresh osteochondral allografts for posttraumatic knee defects. Clin Orthop Relat Res 2005;(435):79–87.
20. Brittberg M, Anders L, Anders N, et al. Treatment of deep cartilage defects in the knee with autologous chondrocyte transplantation. N Engl J Med 1994;331(14):889–95.
21. Mithofer K, Peterson L, Mandelbaum BR, et al. Articular cartilage repair in soccer players with autologous chondrocyte transplantation: functional outcome and return to competition. Am J Sports Med 2005;33(11):1639–46.
22. Mithofer K, Minas T, Peterson L, et al. Functional outcome of knee articular cartilage repair in adolescent athletes. Am J Sports Med 2005;33(8):1147–53.
23. Peterson L, Minas T, Brittberg M, et al. Two- to 9-year outcome after autologous chondrocyte transplantation of the knee. Clin Orthop Relat Res 2000;(374):212–34.
24. Peterson L, Brittberg M, Kiviranta I, et al. Autologous chondrocyte transplantation. Biomechanics and long-term durability. Am J Sports Med 2002;30(1):2–12.
25. Henderson I, Gui J, Lavigne P. Autologous chondrocyte implantation: natural history of postimplantation periosteal hypertrophy and effects of repair-site debridement on outcome. Arthroscopy 2006;22(12):1318–1324.e1.
26. Wood JJ, Malek MA, Frassica FJ, et al. Autologous cultured chondrocytes: adverse events reported to the United States Food and Drug Administration. J Bone Joint Surg Am 2006;88(3):503–7.
27. Saris DB, Vanlauwe J, Victor J, et al. Characterized chondrocyte implantation results in better structural repair when treating symptomatic cartilage defects of the knee in a randomized controlled trial versus microfracture. Am J Sports Med 2008;36(2):235–46.
28. Hoemann CD, Hurtig M, Rossomacha E, et al. Chitosan-glycerol phosphate/blood implants improve hyaline cartilage repair in ovine microfracture defects. J Bone Joint Surg Am 2005;87(12):2671–86.
29. Hoemann CD, Sun J, McKee MD, et al. Chitosan-glycerol phosphate/blood implants elicit hyaline cartilage repair integrated with porous subchondral bone in microdrilled rabbit defects. Osteoarthritis Cartilage 2007;15(1):78–89.
30. Marchand C, Chen G, Tran-Khanh N, et al. Microdrilled cartilage defects treated with thrombin-solidified chitosan/blood implant regenerate a more hyaline, stable, and structurally integrated osteochondral unit compared to drilled controls. Tissue Eng Part A 2012;18(5–6):508–19.
31. Wang DA, Varghese S, Sharma B, et al. Multifunctional chondroitin sulphate for cartilage tissue-biomaterial integration. Nat Mater 2007;6(5):385–92.
32. Milano G, Sanna Passino E, Deriu L, et al. The effect of platelet rich plasma combined with microfractures on the treatment of chondral defects: an experimental study in a sheep model. Osteoarthritis Cartilage 2010;18(7):971–80.
33. Fortier LA, Potter HG, Rickey EJ, et al. Concentrated bone marrow aspirate improves full-thickness cartilage repair compared with microfracture in the equine model. J Bone Joint Surg Am 2010;92(10):1927–37.
34. Saw KY, Hussin P, Loke SC, et al. Articular cartilage regeneration with autologous marrow aspirate and hyaluronic Acid: an experimental study in a goat model. Arthroscopy 2009;25(12):1391–400.
35. Serra R, Johnson M, Filvaroff EH, et al. Expression of a truncated, kinase-defective TGF-beta type II receptor in mouse skeletal tissue promotes terminal chondrocyte differentiation and osteoarthritis. J Cell Biol 1997;139(2):541–52.
36. Trippel SB. Growth factor actions on articular cartilage. J Rheumatol Suppl 1995;43:129–32.

37. Bonassar LJ, Grodzinsky AJ, Frank EH, et al. The effect of dynamic compression on the response of articular cartilage to insulin-like growth factor-I. J Orthop Res 2001;19(1):11–7.
38. Tavera C, Abribat T, Reboul P, et al. IGF and IGF-binding protein system in the synovial fluid of osteoarthritic and rheumatoid arthritic patients. Osteoarthritis Cartilage 1996;4(4):263–74.
39. Sailor LZ, Hewick RM, Morris EA. Recombinant human bone morphogenetic protein-2 maintains the articular chondrocyte phenotype in long-term culture. J Orthop Res 1996;14(6):937–45.
40. Baums MH, Heidrich G, Schultz W, et al. Autologous chondrocyte transplantation for treating cartilage defects of the talus. J Bone Joint Surg Am 2006;88(2): 303–8.
41. Bartlett W, Skinner JA, Gooding CR, et al. Autologous chondrocyte implantation versus matrix-induced autologous chondrocyte implantation for osteochondral defects of the knee: a prospective, randomised study. J Bone Joint Surg Br 2005;87(5):640–5.
42. Filardo G, Kon E, Di Martino A, et al. Arthroscopic second-generation autologous chondrocyte implantation: a prospective 7-year follow-up study. Am J Sports Med 2011;39(10):2153–60.
43. Giza E, Sullivan M, Ocel D, et al. Matrix-induced autologous chondrocyte implantation of talus articular defects. Foot Ankle Int 2010;31(9):747–53.
44. Giannini S, Buda R, Vannini F, et al. Arthroscopic autologous chondrocyte implantation in osteochondral lesions of the talus: surgical technique and results. Am J Sports Med 2008;36(5):873–80.
45. Giannini S, Buda R, Vannini F, et al. One-step bone marrow-derived cell transplantation in talar osteochondral lesions. Clin Orthop Relat Res 2009;467(12): 3307–20.
46. Sun Y, Feng Y, Zhang CQ, et al. The regenerative effect of platelet-rich plasma on healing in large osteochondral defects. Int Orthop 2010;34(4):589–97.
47. Cook JL. Tissue engineering approaches to cartilage repair in AOFAS. San Diego (CA). 2012.
48. Lu Y, Dhanaraj S, Wang Z, et al. Minced cartilage without cell culture serves as an effective intraoperative cell source for cartilage repair. J Orthop Res 2006;24(6): 1261–70.
49. Frisbie DD, Lu Y, Kawcak CE, et al. In vivo evaluation of autologous cartilage fragment-loaded scaffolds implanted into equine articular defects and compared with autologous chondrocyte implantation. Am J Sports Med 2009;37(Suppl 1): 71S–80S.
50. Cole BJ, Farr J, Winalski CS, et al. Outcomes after a single-stage procedure for cell-based cartilage repair: a prospective clinical safety trial with 2-year follow-up. Am J Sports Med 2011;39(6):1170–9.
51. Mithoefer K, McAdams TR, Scopp JM, et al. Emerging options for treatment of articular cartilage injury in the athlete. Clin Sports Med 2009;28(1):25–40.
52. Adams SB, Yao JQ, Schon LC. Particulated juvenile articular cartilage allograft transplantation for osteochondral lesions of the Talus. Tech Foot Ankle Surg 2011;10(2):92–8.
53. Temple TH. Cartilage matrix for talus OCD in AOFAS Summer Meeting. San Diego (CA). 2012.
54. De Mattei M, Fini M, Setti S, et al. Proteoglycan synthesis in bovine articular cartilage explants exposed to different low-frequency low-energy pulsed electromagnetic fields. Osteoarthritis Cartilage 2007;15(2):163–8.

55. De Mattei M, Pasello M, Pellati A, et al. Effects of electromagnetic fields on proteoglycan metabolism of bovine articular cartilage explants. Connect Tissue Res 2003;44(3–4):154–9.
56. Fini M, Giavaresi G, Torricelli P, et al. Pulsed electromagnetic fields reduce knee osteoarthritic lesion progression in the aged Dunkin Hartley guinea pig. J Orthop Res 2005;23(4):899–908.
57. Benazzo F, Cadossi M, Cavani F, et al. Cartilage repair with osteochondral autografts in sheep: effect of biophysical stimulation with pulsed electromagnetic fields. J Orthop Res 2008;26(5):631–42.
58. Zorzi C, Dall'Oca C, Cadossi R, et al. Effects of pulsed electromagnetic fields on patients' recovery after arthroscopic surgery: prospective, randomized and double-blind study. Knee Surg Sports Traumatol Arthrosc 2007;15(7):830–4.
59. Dragoo JL, Samimi B, Zhu M, et al. Tissue-engineered cartilage and bone using stem cells from human infrapatellar fat pads. J Bone Joint Surg Br 2003;85(5):740–7.
60. Grande DA, Mason J, Light E, et al. Stem cells as platforms for delivery of genes to enhance cartilage repair. J Bone Joint Surg Am 2003;85(Suppl 2):111–6.

Osteochondral Lesions of the Talus: Size, Age, and Predictors of Outcomes

Premjit Pete S. Deol, DO[a], Daniel J. Cuttica, DO[b],
William Bret Smith, DO, MS[c], Gregory C. Berlet, MD[d],*

KEYWORDS

- Osteochondritis dissecans • Osteochondral lesion • Talus • Cartilage

KEY POINTS

- Treatment of osteochondral lesions of the talus (OLTs) is an evolving area, with generally 85% good to excellent results with current techniques.
- Additional therapies are continuing to evolve to modify the biological healing response to improve outcomes.
- Future direction of OLT treatment will likely rely on maximizing the combined effects of biological, chemical, and structural therapies to provide the most reliable treatment options.
- Lesion size, lesion containment, and patient age play a role in treatment outcomes, and these variables need to be considered to guide the surgeon in decision making.

INTRODUCTION

Osteochondral lesions of the talus (OLTs) offer a significant challenge to the foot and ankle specialist. OLTs can cause pain and decreased function in our patients. Many questions remain about the nature of these injuries. There is a continuous search to understand more about this unique disease.

Isolating prognostic factors for patients with OLTs has been one of our main research goals over the past decade. This research has led us to explore the role of lesion size, the meaning of the marrow edema, age of the patient, containment of the lesion, and the many methods of creating a stable cartilage cap.

The size of the lesion and extent of edema are intertwined. Often the qualitative information received about a patient with an OLT is the size of the lesion on magnetic resonance imaging (MRI) (**Figs. 1** and **2**). On MRI, the articular defect must be clearly distinguished from the edema halo surrounding the lesion. The early signs of healing

[a] Panorama Orthopedics and Spine Center, 660 Golden Ridge Road, Suite 250, Golden, CO 80401, USA; [b] The Orthopaedic Foot and Ankle Center of Washington D.C., 2922 Falls Church, VA 22042, USA; [c] Moore Orthopedics, 104 Saluda Pointe Drive, Lexington, SC 29072, USA; [d] Orthopedic Foot and Ankle Center, 300 Polaris Parkway, Suite 2000, Westerville, OH 43082, USA
* Corresponding author.
E-mail address: ofacresearch@orthofootankle.com

Foot Ankle Clin N Am 18 (2013) 13–34
http://dx.doi.org/10.1016/j.fcl.2012.12.010
1083-7515/13/$ – see front matter © 2013 Elsevier Inc. All rights reserved.

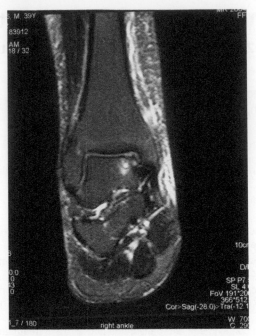

Fig. 1. Coronal MRI image of an OLT.

include decreased edema response, but a stable cartilage cap is necessary for the permanent resolution of this edema. We believe that the clinical symptoms of pain can be correlated with the edema response to articular injury.

In this article, our research on OLTs is summarized, the orthopedic literature is reviewed, and the direction of future research and treatment trends is discussed.

Historical Perspective

Kappis originally described OLTs in 1922.[1] Before his description of the process in the ankle, Konig in 1888[2] defined the term osteochondritis dissecans to describe

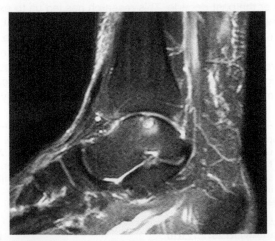

Fig. 2. Sagittal MRI image of an OLT.

a process of loose body formation associated with articular cartilage and subchondral bone fracture in the hip and knee. In 1959, Berndt and Harty developed a staging system based on radiographic and surgical parameters, which has become the most widely used system of classification for OLTs (**Table 1**).[3] The premise of their classification centered on the OLT and whether there was displacement of the fragment.

Since the advent of computed tomography (CT), MRI, and arthroscopy, the limitations of the Berndt and Harty classification have been shown.

Numerous other classification systems have been suggested.[4–9] These classifications looked to improve on the original classification in hopes of improving treatment protocols and outcomes and enabling a more accurate discussion so that like lesions are being accurately compared.

Predictors of Clinical Outcomes

Numerous studies have shown that treatment outcomes for OLTs using a variety of surgical techniques have a roughly 85% efficacy rate. Ideally, as large an improvement as possible on the outcomes in those patients is desired. An attempt to identify and stratify those predictors of outcomes would offer the foot and ankle surgeon an improved treatment algorithm to offer their patient. Numerous parameters have been studied to look for predictors of outcomes. These parameters have included age, sex, duration of symptoms, and location and size of lesion. Most studies have supplied some, but limited, data in predicting patient outcomes.

CURRENT TREATMENT CONCEPTS
Nonoperative Treatment

Initial treatment options for chronic OLTs or acute on chronic lesions often begin with nonoperative measures, because many of these are found incidentally on imaging. An acute osteochondral fracture with displacement is a contraindication to nonoperative treatment. Nonoperative treatment involves immobilization such as casting or prefabricated walking boots, nonsteroidal antiinflammatory medications, bracing, corticosteroid injections, and activity modification.

The results of nonoperative treatment are variable. In a large meta-analysis including 32 studies,[10] nonoperative treatment produced good or excellent results in 45% of patients. Shearer and colleagues[11] assessed the clinical outcomes of 35 ankles with stage 5 OLTs treated nonoperatively. Fifty-four percent of patients in this study had a good or excellent outcome at an average of 38 months after treatment. There were 13 ankles that had mild degenerative changes at final follow-up; however, the presence of any degenerative changes did not correlate with clinical symptoms. The investigators concluded that nonoperative treatment of these lesions is a viable option, with little or no risk of developing significant osteoarthritis.

Table 1 Berndt and Harty classification system	
Stage 1	Small subchondral compression fracture
Stage 2	Partially detached fragment
Stage 3	Completely detached without displacement
Stage 4	Detached and displaced within the joint

Data from Berndt AL, Harty M. Transchondral fractures (osteochondritis dissecans) of the talus. J Bone Joint Surg Am 1959;41:988–1020.

More recently, hyaluronate injections and platelet-rich plasma (PRP) have been described as a nonoperative option for OLTs. A prospective study showed improved scores in pain and function in 15 patients, after 3 weekly injections of hyaluronate, which lasted for 6 months.[12] In another study, Mei-Dan and colleagues[13] compared the short-term clinical efficacy of hyaluronate injections with PRP injections in 32 patients. Both groups had improvements in pain and function at final follow-up of 6 months; however, the PRP group had significantly better clinical outcomes compared with the hyaluronate group.

Operative Treatment

Operative treatment is indicated in those patients with symptomatic, focal OLTs that have failed nonoperative treatment, and in those with an acute, displaced fragment. Current operative treatment options include open reduction and internal fixation of displaced fragments. For osteochondral defects, contemporary options include marrow stimulation techniques, osteochondral autograft or allograft transfer (OATS), or autologous chondrocyte implantation (ACI).

Marrow stimulation

Marrow stimulation techniques include drilling or microfracture and are often considered first-line treatment. This procedure is usually performed arthroscopically, and consists of excision of the OLT to a stable cartilage border. The subchondral bone is penetrated via microfracture or drilling, which causes the subchondral bone to bleed and to produce fibrocartilage formation at the OLT.[14,15]

There have been multiple studies evaluating the effectiveness of marrow stimulation techniques for treatment of OLTs, with good to excellent outcomes, ranging from 65% to 90%.[4,5,10,16–24]

Tol and colleagues,[10] in their large meta-analysis, evaluated treatment options for OLTs. These options included nonoperative treatment, excision of the OLT, excision and curettage, and excision of the OLT with marrow stimulation. The highest average success rate was in the excision and marrow stimulation group, with 85% of patients having good or excellent results, followed by excision and curettage, with 78% of patients with favorable results.

Another study[4] evaluated the long-term results after arthroscopic marrow stimulation of OLTs. The investigators reported 72% good or excellent results, at an average of 71 months follow-up. However, this study does provide concern about long-term function, because 35% of patients showed a deterioration of their result over time. Those patients with unstable lesions had inferior clinical outcomes.

Repeat marrow stimulation has been shown to be of benefit in those who have failed a previous procedure. Schuman and colleagues[23] evaluated 38 patients who underwent OLT curettage and drilling, including 22 primary procedures and 16 revision procedures. These investigators reported 86% and 75% good or excellent results in the primary and revision groups, respectively. More recently, the clinical outcomes of 12 patients who underwent repeat arthroscopy and debridement of the OLT were evaluated, with 11 of 12 patients satisfied with their clinical outcome at an average of 5.9 years follow-up.[22] However, Robinson and colleagues[21] showed that the results of repeat arthroscopic marrow stimulation in patients who failed a previous procedure can be disappointing.

For OLTs that have an intact cartilage cap, retrograde drilling has been described to prevent violation of the intact cartilage cap. Taranow and colleagues[25] retrospectively reviewed the results of 16 patients who underwent retrograde drilling for medial OLTs, reporting an 81% patient satisfaction rate. Of the few patients who were unsatisfied,

3 were workers' compensation cases. Kono and colleagues[19] compared retrograde drilling with transmalleolar drilling in 30 patients and found significantly better outcomes in the retrograde drilling group. Most recently, the results of retrograde drilling using a novel cannulated drilling system have been described.[26] The investigators reported favorable results, similar to other studies. However, the use of a cannulated drilling system simplified the procedure, maximizing time and accuracy when performing retrograde drilling.

Several variables may be predictive of clinical outcome after marrow stimulation, in particular, OLT size, patient age, cystic nature of the lesion, and containment of the lesion.

Lesion size may be the most important predictor. Various studies have shown that lesion size affects clinical outcome, with size larger than 1.5 cm^2 associated with inferior outcomes.[27–29] This situation is most likely because larger OLTs have been shown to cause significant changes in the contact characteristics of the ankle joint.[30]

Chuckpaiwong and colleagues[28] found a strong correlation between lesion size and clinical outcome, having excellent results in patients with OLT sizes less than 15 mm. Other factors such as increasing age, higher body mass index (calculated as weight in kilograms divided by the square of height in meters), history of trauma, and presence of osteophytes negatively affected outcome. In another study, Choi and colleagues[27] evaluated 120 ankles that underwent arthroscopic marrow stimulation for OLTs to determine prognostic factors for clinical outcome. These investigators concluded that OLTs larger than 150 mm^2 were associated with poor outcomes after treatment. Other factors such as age, duration of symptoms, trauma, associated lesions, and location of lesions had no association with outcome.

In the largest study, Cuttica and colleagues[29] retrospectively reviewed the subjective clinical outcomes of 130 patients after marrow stimulation for OLTs. Multiple variables were analyzed, including patient age, body mass index, history of trauma, OLT location, cystic nature of the lesion, containment of the lesion, and history of trauma. Through an extensive statistical analysis, the investigators found that OLT size greater than 1.5 cm^2 was the most important predictor of a poor outcome. Uncontained OLTs and age were also shown to contribute to overall outcome.

Patient age may also be a contributing factor. Various reports have shown that a younger age is often associated with better outcomes.[20,29] Kumai and colleagues[20] reported better outcomes after arthroscopic drilling in patients younger than 30 years. Deol and colleagues[31] performed a retrospective review in an attempt to determine if age played a role in outcomes. In their study, all patients treated for an OLT with marrow stimulation who were younger than 18 years had a good or excellent outcome. The investigators attributed the results to the rich microvascular supply within the subchondral zone in patients with open physes and in those recently achieving skeletal maturity.

However, other reports have shown that age does not play a role.[17,32] Becher and Thermann showed that the clinical results in patients older than 50 years were similar to those in younger patients after microfracture.[17] A more recent study of 173 ankles showed that increasing age was not an independent risk factor for a poor clinical outcome after arthroscopic treatment. However, older patients were less likely to have a history of trauma and had a longer duration of symptoms.[32]

The containment of the OLT is another factor that may play a role in overall outcome. OLTs that are contained have a stable periphery, which protects the fibrocartilage that forms at the treated OLT. However, an uncontained lesion involves the shoulder of the talar dome and lacks a stable border of cartilage at the site of microfracture (**Fig. 3**). Without a stable rim, the protective border is lost and the treated area is subjected

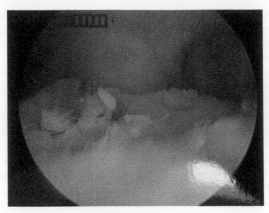

Fig. 3. Arthroscopic image of an uncontained OLT.

to greater stresses, making a stable area of fibrocartilage formation less likely. This finding is supported by Cuttica and colleagues,[29] who showed that an uncontained OLT was an independent predictor of a poor outcome. This is the only study showing that lesion containment plays a role in outcomes.

Cystic OLTs have been shown by some investigators to have a negative impact on outcomes, whereas others have shown that the cystic nature of the lesion has no impact. Two separate studies showed that treatment of small cystic OLTs with marrow stimulation yielded satisfactory results.[5,18] However, others argue that cystic lesions need to be treated with bone grafting.[4,33] In addition, Robinson and colleagues[21] had a 53% incidence of poor outcomes after marrow stimulation for cystic OLTs.

OSTEOCHONDRAL AUTOGRAFT/ALLOGRAFT TRANSFER SYSTEM

Osteochondral autografts can be used to treat larger OLTs as the initial procedure, or for revision procedures that have failed marrow stimulation. The OLT is replaced with an osteochondral plug or multiple plugs, with a hyaline cartilage surface and bone-to-bone healing of the plug with the talus. This technique has the theoretic advantage of restoring hyaline cartilage at the OLT. The autogenous graft is typically taken from a nonweight-bearing portion of the ipsilateral knee or talus, and is placed flush with the articular surface. Perpendicular access to the OLT is required, which often necessitates the use of a malleolar osteotomy.

The results after OATS have been favorable in many studies.[34–39] In the largest study, Hangody and colleagues[36] reported the results of 63 patients with a mosaic-plasty autogenous osteochondral transplant for OLTs, with an average lesion size of 1 cm², and an average of 5.8 years follow-up. The donor site was the superomedial edge of the medial femoral condyle. Fifty-eight patients had good or excellent results at final follow-up. There was a 3% incidence of donor site morbidity.

More recently, a prospective randomized study compared the clinical outcomes after chondroplasty, microfracture, and OATS in patients with OLTs with 2 years follow-up. Results showed no difference in outcomes between the procedures at final follow-up, suggesting that there may be no benefit of OATS over chondroplasty or microfracture.[40] However, this study consisted of a small sample size of only 30 patients, with short-term follow-up.

Donor site morbidity is a potential complication of OATS procedures. The incidence has been low in several studies.[34,36,41,42] However, 1 study reported the incidence of donor site morbidity to be as high as 36%, with no significant difference in terms of the harvest method or number of grafts obtained.[43]

The concern over donor site morbidity, as well as large, deep lesions or shoulder lesions that would make autograft use difficult, has led to the use of fresh allograft in many cases. In such cases, a CT scan is used to determine the dimensions of the native talus, which are sent to a tissue bank to find a matching talus. It can take up to several months to find a match. Once a matching talus is obtained, it should be implanted within 14 days to maximize chondrocyte viability.[44]

Multiple studies have shown the effectiveness of fresh talar allograft for OLTs.[45–50] El Rashidi and colleagues[47] reported on the use of fresh talar allograft in 38 patients, with an average of 37.7 months follow-up. There were 28 patients with good, very good, or excellent results, with only 4 graft failures. Berlet and colleagues[46] conducted a prospective evaluation of 8 patients with shoulder lesions treated with fresh talar allograft, with an average of 48 months follow-up. All patients had improvement in pain and functional scores at final follow-up. However, radiographic lucencies were noted at the graft-host interface at final follow-up in 5 patients. Raikin[50] prospectively evaluated fresh osteochondral allografting for large-volume (>3000 mm^3) cystic lesions, with a minimum of 2 years follow-up in 15 patients. There was an 87% graft survival at 2 years, and 73% good or excellent results. There were 2 failures, which went on to arthrodesis.

Potential disadvantages of allograft include the low risk for disease transmission, immunologic reaction to the graft, and long-term time interval for graft incorporation.

1. A 16-year-old gymnast who has had 6 months of pain. A 150-mm posteromedial lesion is present. Not on the shoulder. She is able to perform, but does so with pain. It is 4 months before her state championships.
   a. In a high caliber athlete participating in a hallmark event, indications for competition are restricted to those who are functional and at low-risk for additional injury. In this scenario, without shoulder involvement or a cystic component, the athlete should be counseled to the relatively low potential of additional injury. Upon completion of the state championship, a treatment regimen should be initiated. If this patient should fail nonoperative treatment, treatment via arthroscopy and microfracture would be indicated. Although this is a large OLT, because of the patient's young age and containment of the OLT, she has a high likelihood of a good outcome following microfracture.
2. A 39-year-old accountant, with a 2 × 3 cm cystic lesion. It is asymptomatic, centro-lateral and has an intact cartilage surface on MRI.
   a. The likelihood of progression is low but must be followed closely clinically and with serial imaging. Initial treatment of observation must be abandoned if the lesion becomes symptomatic or increases. Arthroscopically-assisted retrograde drilling and bone grafting of the cystic region is a technically rewarding approach, as long as the cartilage cap remains intact. If the overlying cartilage is violated upon arthroscopic investigation, open bone grafting with subsequent chondrocyte implantation would serve to address the bony void and cartilage defect.
3. A 30-year-old professional soccer player. He tripped 1 year ago, and has undergone a previous arthroscopy and marrow stimulation. There is a lot of surrounding edema on MRI and the CT shows complete loss of the cartilage surface. He is symptomatic and it is the middle of the season with 2 months left to play.

a. Professional athletes require a unique balance between maximizing functional improvement, minimizing invasive intervention while expediting a return to play. This scenario highlights the need for temporary symptom management potentially with corticosteroid or viscoscupplementation injections, bracing and possibly platelet rich plasma to control short-term symptoms. More definitive treatment could then be taken on during the off-season with chondrocyte grafting using autologous or allograft tissues sources.

4. A 20-year-old construction worker. He fell one year ago off a ladder and sustained an acute osteochondral fracture treated operatively with a resorbable pin fixation. He is symptomatic. The lesion is posteromedial, involved the shoulder of the talus and measures 2 × 2 cm.

   a. The challenge in treating lesions along the shoulder of the talus involve maintaining cartilage repair stability. If the underlying fracture component is well healed with an intact subchondral plate, an initial attempt at microfracture would be warranted given the patient's age. Because of the large size of the OLT and its uncontained nature, the patient should be counseled that there is a high likelihood of a poor outcome with microfracture. Failure of microfracturing would then necessitate consideration for autologous chondrocyte grafting or possible an osteochondral allograft implant.

   b. I would have to give serious consideration to osteochondral allograft implantation in this scenario as an initial procedure. Of course the suspicion that this is likely a workers compensation case might temper my enthusiasm.

5. A 28-year-old recreational squash player. Prior arthroscopy, unknown procedure and no documentation of the lesion or treatment. A 150-mm^2 centrolateral shoulder lesion with a 0.5 cm × 1.0 cm "kissing" tibial lesion. He wants to continue to play squash.

   a. Given that this young, active patient's index procedure is unknown, treatment warrants an attempt at marrow stimulation if he is symptomatic. Ferkel and several other authors have documented good success with repeat microfracturing and marrow stimulation techniques following initial surgical failure. Both lesions should be addressed at the same setting. Failure of microfracturing would then suggest a chondrocyte implantation approach be considered.

6. A 140-mm lesion, in a 50-year-old female recreational golfer. She has constant pain, is able to play but wants to continue a few more months of playing before definitive treatment.

   a. Contained lesions without impending subchondral collapse are at a relatively low risk of sudden progression. If symptom management is necessary for a short period, consideration should be made for bracing and/or a corticosteroid injection. Once the patient is able pursue definitive treatment, an initial attempt at marrow stimulation techniques should be contemplated.

AUTOLOGOUS CHONDROCYTE IMPLANTATION

ACI involves transplantation of cultured chondrocytes into the OLT, which is sealed by a periosteal patch. It involves 2 separate surgical procedures. The first procedure involves harvest of cartilage from the talus or femoral condyle. The chondrocytes from the harvested cartilage are cultured in a laboratory for 2 to 3 weeks. At the second procedure, the OLT is debrided, a periosteal patch is taken from the distal tibia and sutured over the lesion, and the cultured chondrocytes are injected into the OLT beneath the periosteal patch. In an effort to decrease any donor site morbidity, the detached chondral fragment or margins from the OLT have been used as an alternative for cartilage harvest.[51]

ACI has been shown to have successful outcomes in multiple retrospective studies.[52–56] Nam and colleagues[55] reported a prospective case series in 11 patients with an average of 38 months follow-up. At final follow-up, there were 9 patients with good or excellent results, and 2 with fair results. Ten of the patients underwent a second-look arthroscopy and all had complete coverage of the OLT. However, there was a 20% incidence of graft hypertrophy. The long-term results after ACI have been evaluated by Giannini and colleagues.[53] At an average of 119 months follow-up, 10 patients had improved American Orthopaedic Foot and Ankle Society scores from 37.9 to 92.7 at final follow-up. A recent review by Wood and colleagues[57] noted a 3.8% incidence of complications after ACI, with the most common reported events being graft failure, delamination, and graft hypertrophy.

Recently, matrix-induced ACI (MACI) for OLTs has been used. MACI modifies the ACI technique by using a porcine collagen membrane carrier for the chondrocytes, which is secured to the lesion with fibrin glue. Possible advantages of this method include reducing operative time, eliminating the need for a periosteal patch, and reducing the likelihood of postoperative complications such as graft hypertrophy or leakage of chondrocytes from the periosteal patch. Early studies have been encouraging,[58,59] although this procedure is not available in the United States.

TALAR OSTEOCHONDRAL LESIONS

The treatment of OLTs continues to represent a difficult and challenging issue within the foot and ankle community. Its treatment has continued to evolve over the past several decades with the exploration of lesions and treatment variables associated within different patient populations. As our independent research has shown over the past several years, specific characteristics of these lesions and patients can potentially assist in improving the quality of treatment outcomes. The importance of lesion size, patient age, and host response are key characteristics at the heart of ongoing research into osteochondral lesions and may lead to the development of an algorithm for the treatment of all OLTs.

SIZE

A feature of osteochondral lesions that has been shown to be of significance is the size of lesions, particularly with response to surgical treatment.[27,28,60] Our research corroborates previous publications showing improved surgical outcomes after bone marrow stimulation for those OLTs smaller than 1.5 mm^2.[29] The potential limitations in healing for larger size lesions have yet to be established. This situation may represent an inherent limitation in the host healing response across a broad surface area, suggesting a potential maximal threshold beyond which a distribution of nutrient and substrates is not possible.

The challenge in treating these larger lesions is to establish an appropriate local environment that will allow induction of therapeutic factors and an appropriate response of locally contained cellular elements to stimulate healing. A critical factor in healing is the abnormal chondrocytes contained within osteochondral lesions, which may not be receptive to stimulation. Koch and colleagues[61] reported an overall decrease in chondrocytes with thinning of the subchondral plate in osteochondral lesions when compared with normal samples. Histologic analysis reveals that the initial changes within the core of the lesion begin with bone necrosis or subchondral fracture, often being replaced with cartilage without identifiable bone trabeculae.[62] New research into the direct stimulation of these cellular elements and development of appropriate scaffolds over which to bridge these larger defects may prove to be beneficial in making lesion size less problematic.

Ultrasound

The use of ultrasound has been extensively studied within orthopedics for its ability to facilitate healing. Although primarily known for its reported acceleration of healing in acute fractures and nonunited fractures when used in low-intensity pulsed applications, its potential benefits in cartilage repair have only recently been identified.[63–66] Xiao-lin and colleagues[67] reported that low-intensity pulsed ultrasound had therapeutic effects on the gross appearance and histologic grades of osteochondral lesions induced within rabbit models. The cellular processes of inducing mature chondrocytes to upregulate matrix gene expression of the aggrecan gene and proteoglycan/chondroitin sulfate synthesis are well documented.[68–71] It has been proposed that ultrasound may work to enhance cartilage matrix formation and maintain chondrocyte differentiation through transforming growth factor β (TGF-β) mediation of human mesenchymal stem cells mesenchymal stem cells (MSCs).[72] The process of ultrasound stimulation also results in an increase in production of vascular endothelial growth factor, fibroblast growth factor, and interleukin 8, all of which are necessary for angiogenesis.[73,74] The direct induction of locally contained chondrocytes and OLTs with low-intensity pulsed ultrasound may help to surpass the critical healing threshold of 1.5 mm^2 with OLTs.

Electrical/Electromagnetic Stimulation

The application of pulsed electromagnetic direct current has also been examined for its potential role in osteochondral injuries. Numerous in vitro investigations have supported the efficacy of electrical stimulation in chondrogenesis.[75–77] Lippello and colleagues[78] reported that direct stimulation on osteochondral lesions of differing sizes improved the quality of repaired articular cartilage. Biochemical analysis of bone and cartilage treated with electrical stimulation has shown an increased expression of numerous molecular signaling agents, including bone morphogenic proteins (BMPs) 2, 4, 5, 6, and 7.[79,80] The proposed cellular response to electrical stimulation induces enhanced differentiation of mesenchymal precursor cells and a proliferation of chondrocytes.[81,82] The application of electrical stimulation to osteochondral lesions has not been shown to have a minimum effective area, although the available literature is limited. Ongoing research should help to determine the potential future efficacy of pulsed electromagnetic direct current treatment in OLTs, particular with larger lesions.[83]

Tissue Scaffolds

Although the quality of cartilage repair is vital to ensure good clinical results, the quantity of cartilage may be even more critical with larger lesions. In larger lesions, there is concern with the poor cartilage-to-cartilage integration that has been witnessed histologically and is believed to be caused by a paucity of structural bonding within the defect.[84] The use of tissue scaffolds over which chondrocytes can be regenerated may be critical in replicating the native osteochondral interface and in crossing the size barrier.

The challenges of developing constructs that improve tissue implant integration are dependent on finding a sufficient scaffold over which to allow growth.[84,85] Various materials, both natural and synthetic, have been investigated to identify ideal pore size, geometry, mechanical properties, and biocompatibility.[86–88] It is believed that the use of these tissue scaffolds will improve functional outcomes through a more uniform distribution of grafted chondrocytes, reduced cellular graft leakage, and controlled overgrowth of regenerated cartilage.[89] The deposition of cultured cells within three-dimensional scaffolds may represent an ability to fulfill the biological, mechanical, and architectural obligations necessary for successful osteochondral repair in large OLTs.

Whether the issues inherent to healing large OLTs are related to specific size limitations, to the quality of the tissue regenerated, or to a deficiency in the quantity of reparative tissue remains unclear. Most likely, a combination of treatment strategies is necessary to overcome the issues related to lesion size.

EDEMA

A unique imaging characteristic of osteochondral lesions often identified on MRI is bony edema immediately adjacent to the area of injury. The prognostic significance of edema has until recently been relatively unclear. Our research has shown that improved clinical symptoms postoperatively correlate with a lower intensity of edema on MRI.[90] However, it is still unclear how the development and resolution of edema correlate with its intensity and extent of involvement within the talus. Identifying factors that relate to increased bony edema may help to expand the horizon of clinical treatment options used in the treatment of OLTs with significant adjacent bony edema, leading to improved clinical results.

Viscosupplementation

One of the postulated mechanisms for the development of talar edema relates to an inducible inflammatory cascade. It has been shown that an intra-articular influx of inflammatory and proteolytic factors occurs after injury or surgical trauma.[91] This cascade is likely regulated by an angiogenic process, resulting in an influx of vascular channels between the tidemark and osteochondral junction, allowing angiogenic factors from chondrocytes and the subchondral bone to perpetuate inflammation, edema, and destructive changes.[92–94] The volume and intensity of edema may therefore correlate with the severity of this intrinsic inflammatory response and likely influence the degree of patient symptoms.

If edema is primarily attributable to cellular and inflammatory mediators, the potential benefit of viscosupplementation becomes clearer as a treatment option. The documented benefits of viscosupplementation include its effects as an antiinflammatory, chondroprotective, analgesic, and anabolic/anticatabolic agent.[95] Its direct and long-term benefits within the ankle are not well published, although the reported benefit of hyaluronic acid in the knee has been well documented.[96] The study of viscosupplementation within the ankle for the treatment of osteochondral lesions has primarily been limited to animal models and individual physician experience.[91]

A primary barrier in the United States to identifying potential benefits of viscosupplementation with hyaluronic acid in the ankle is its limited approval by the Food and Drug Administration to the knee only. Recently, several studies have reported potentially promising results for the possible future expansion of its indications for destructive cartilage processes within the ankle.[97–99] With the current limitations in the available literature for use in foot and ankle conditions, the use of viscosupplementation continues to struggle to find its place in current treatment algorithms until more high-quality publications become available.

Navigation

An alternative hypothesis for the development of bony edema associated with osteochondral lesions postulated by van Dijk and colleagues[100] focuses on the violation of the overlying subchondral bone. With violation of the subchondral plate, spontaneous resolution of bone edema can be impaired or inhibited because of continued extravasation of pressurized joint fluid into the defect, leading to increased intraosseous pressure.[101,102] A similar phenomenon has been reported to occur within the hip during early stages of osteonecrosis, when symptomatic patients reporting hip pain show an increase in hydrostatic bone marrow pressure with histologic correlation of increased bone marrow edema.[103,104]

Successful treatment of osteonecrosis of the hip with core decompression has been shown to reduce bone marrow edema within the hip, leading to improved clinical results.[103] An association between persistent talar edema and pain associated with osteochondral lesions has also been supported in numerous publications, including our own research.[90,105] Although a similar phenomenon within the talus requires continued investigation, this information may help us address our patients with painful and persistent talar edema using selective talar decompression techniques.

A challenge with effective decompression for the talus is gaining access to the edematous area in a safe manner without creating additional injury. The application of navigation and computer-assisted surgery to address intra-articular disease of the knee has been well documented, particularly with retrograde techniques for osteochondral lesions.[106] Several publications applying navigation to disease of the ankle and hindfoot have also sparked greater interest in its applications within the foot and ankle community.[107,108] The continued expansion of this technology to OLTs may represent a more accurate and precise manner to potentially address increased intraosseous pressure and persistent talar edema in symptomatic patients.

Resurfacing

The long-term prognosis and potential complications of talar edema adjacent to osteochondral lesions is not well defined. The intensity and extent of edema surrounding these lesions may have a critical threshold beyond which their ability to heal may be compromised.[101,102] As the associated subchondral bone is damaged, osteolysis can occur and lead to local osteonecrosis, bone resorption, and formation of lytic areas.[109–114] These larger edematous areas may therefore benefit from a more aggressive treatment approach to avoid potential future collapse and destruction of the joint.

In the development of osteoarthritis, the articular cartilage undergoes progressive thinning and the osteochondral junction is insulted by an advancing wave of ossification.[92] It is unclear whether this process can be halted with excision of the diseased areas before its spread across a greater portion of the joint. If a greater intensity and area of bone edema with associated osteochondral injury represents a risk for progressive disease and chondral injury, focal resurfacing may be a consideration to spare the remaining joint. Resurfacing may also have a role in larger lesions because larger lesions had a shift in peak stress toward the lesion, with an overall decrease in ankle contact area, which could lead to progressive deterioration.[115] Although long-term results are unavailable, the development of metal inlay implants represents a promising approach to this challenge.[116,117]

The issues related to talar edema associated with OLTs are a topic that has only recently been highlighted. The characteristics and importance of this edematous response are still being identified. As we gain a greater appreciation of the intensity and extent of talar edema, improved solutions for its treatment and resolution will be made.

AGE

Patient characteristics are a major factor that can influence the success of treatment of OLTs. Youth is generally considered to be a major advantage in the healing of injuries to the osteochondral interface. This finding has been shown in several basic science publications, in which an age-related decline in chondrogenic potential of chondrocytes and chondrogenic stem cells has been seen in both animal and human models.[118,119] The benefits of youth have also been well documented clinically, with improved outcomes in the treatment of osteochondral injuries of the knee in younger patients.[120,121] Our research supports this same finding in lesions of the talus, with patients younger than 18 years showing significantly better outcomes than older patients after microfracture and drilling. These findings suggest that an emphasis be placed on developing strategies that can mimic the biochemical and structural milieu of nonadult patients to potentially improve outcomes.

Platelet Rich Plasma

PRP has gained in popularity over the past decade, with a reported ability to improve intrinsic healing capacity. PRP represents a volume of plasma in which the platelet concentration exceeds normal physiologic levels. This solution, which represents the clot formed in response to an injury, contains an increased concentration of platelet-derived growth factor and TGF-β from α-granules.[122] These growth factors play critical roles in stimulating osteogenesis and chondrogenesis in vivo and are believed to provide a higher dose of growth factors to augment healing.[123,124] Their use in conjunction with ACI has been investigated and shown to be of benefit.[125,126] Although poor literature support exists for the use of PRP for primary treatment of osteochondral lesions, the potential addition of osteogenic and chondrogenic factors to the area of injury may foster an environment similar to those of nonadult patients, who possess a higher potential for healing.

Tissue Engineering

In an older patient population, an augmentation of the natural healing response to mimic younger patients may require the application of advanced tissue engineering techniques. Tissue engineering applies the principles of biological, chemical, and engineering sciences to osteochondral regeneration, focusing on the expansion of cellular sources for repair, providing a platform to allow cellular growth and to ensure a sufficient supply of bioactive molecules that can mediate the repair.[85] Recent advances in tissue engineering have led to the isolation of specific growth factors that may provide a unique method of augmenting the osteochondral healing process. Several growth factors and cytokines have been established as critical to the growth and differentiation of both cartilage and bone, including epidermal growth factor, TGF-β, and insulinlike growth factor.[85,127–129] BMP-2 is of particular interest, because it is involved in the differentiation of MSCs into chondroblasts and osteoblasts.[130] Osteochondral injuries created in an animal model showed accelerated formation of subchondral bone with improved histologic appearance of articular cartilage after the application of recombinant human BMP-2.[130–132] Although many challenges still exist in the potential application of these findings, particularly in delivery and mainte-nance of appropriate therapeutic levels, growth factors represent an exciting future therapeutic option.

MSCs are an area of intense interest within tissue engineering. This progenitor cell source has the potential to differentiate into specific cell lines, which could directly supply bioactive molecules independently to areas of injury. The use of MSCs could allow for relatively unlimited cellular expansion with insignificant donor morbidity at a low cost with ease of availability. Numerous sources of MSCs have been investigated, with those originating from bone marrow aspiration yielding the best chondrogenic and osteogenic potential.[133–135] The implantation of MSCs into osteochondral defects with or without a scaffold has been shown to significantly improve the success of osteochondral repair in numerous animal models.[136–138] The use of MSCs within osteochondral defects should greatly improve longer-term outcomes as the technology, viability and delivery of these cells into the area of injury continues to evolve.

In an effort to capitalize on the chondrogenic potential of nonadult patients, there has also been increased interest in the use of isolated immature chondrocytes. Several commercially available products using scaffold-free, tissue-engineered grafts of living chondrocytes obtained from donor juvenile patients are in development or available for implantation. Initial experience seems to be promising, although longer-term data are still being collected. The specific clinical indications and lesion parameters that might benefit from juvenile chondrocyte implantation still need to be determined.

The evolution of tissue engineering for osteochondral disease will undoubtedly include significant advances in the technology and techniques used in cellular expansion and growth factor synthesis. Low oxygen tension environments, mechanical stimulation, microgravity, and rotating-wall vessels have already been shown to be of benefit in cartilage formation and may represent an important shift in future research.[139–144] The future of treatment of osteochondral lesion is bright and exciting, with a tremendous amount of work still to be done.

SUMMARY

Osteochondral injuries are a challenging but exciting field within orthopedics and the foot and ankle community. Although most patients do well with current treatment strategies for OLTs, those who struggle in their recovery are a population who need to be addressed. The roles of lesion size, edema, and patient age are clear barriers to maximizing patient outcomes across all patient groups. Continued basic science and clinical investigation into these areas could facilitate the development of a treatment algorithm that will foster a reduction of long-term morbidity and an improvement in patient and physician satisfaction.

As this field continues to develop, well-developed research protocols and standardized outcome measures will be necessary to allow effective comparison of outcomes. The parallel challenge of developing and implementing this newer technology in a cost-effective manner will also need to be addressed. The goal of this endeavor will be to apply the most clinically beneficial therapies in the most cost-efficient manner to improve the overall value of orthopedic care, reduce long-term morbidity, and improve quality of life.

REFERENCES

1. Kappis MK. Weitere Beiträge zur traumatisch-mechanischen Entstehung der "spontanen" Knorpelabiosungen. Dtsch Z Chir 1922;171:13–29 [in German].
2. Konig F. Über freie Körper in den Gelenken. Dtsch Z Chir 1888;27:90–109 [in German].
3. Berndt AL, Harty M. Transchondral fractures (osteochondritis dissecans) of the talus. J Bone Joint Surg Am 1959;41:988–1020.

4. Ferkel RD, Zanotti RM, Komenda GA, et al. Arthroscopic treatment of chronic osteochondral lesions of the talus: long-term results. Am J Sports Med 2008; 36(9):1750–62.
5. Loomer R, Fisher C, Lloyd-Smith R, et al. Osteochondral lesions of the talus. Am J Sports Med 1993;21(1):13–9.
6. Pritsch M, Horoshovski H, Farine I. Arthroscopic treatment of osteochondral lesions of the talus. J Bone Joint Surg Am 1986;68(6):862–5.
7. Dipaola JD, Nelson DW, Colville MR. Characterizing osteochondral lesions by magnetic resonance imaging. Arthroscopy 1991;7(1):101–4.
8. Hepple S, Winson IG, Glew D. Osteochondral lesions of the talus: a revised classification. Foot Ankle Int 1999;20(12):789–93.
9. Cheng M, Ferkel RD, Applegate GR. Osteochondral lesion of the talus: a radiologic and surgical comparison. Paper presented at: Annual Meeting of the Academy of Orthopaedic Surgeons. New Orleans, February, 1995.
10. Tol JL, Struijs PA, Bossuyt PM, et al. Treatment strategies in osteochondral defects of the talar dome: a systematic review. Foot Ankle Int 2000;21(2):119–26.
11. Shearer C, Loomer R, Clement D. Nonoperatively managed stage 5 osteochondral talar lesions. Foot Ankle Int 2002;23(7):651–4.
12. Mei-Dan O, Maoz G, Swartzon M, et al. Treatment of osteochondritis dissecans of the ankle with hyaluronic acid injections: a prospective study. Foot Ankle Int 2008;29(12):1171–8.
13. Mei-Dan O, Carmont MR, Laver L, et al. Platelet-rich plasma or hyaluronate in the management of osteochondral lesions of the talus. Am J Sports Med 2012;40(3):534–41.
14. Alford JW, Cole BJ. Cartilage restoration, part 1: basic science, historical perspective, patient evaluation, and treatment options. Am J Sports Med 2005;33(2):295–306.
15. Furukawa T, Eyre DR, Koide S, et al. Biochemical studies on repair cartilage resurfacing experimental defects in the rabbit knee. J Bone Joint Surg Am 1980; 62(1):79–89.
16. Barnes CJ, Ferkel RD. Arthroscopic debridement and drilling of osteochondral lesions of the talus. Foot Ankle Clin 2003;8(2):243–57.
17. Becher C, Thermann H. Results of microfracture in the treatment of articular cartilage defects of the talus. Foot Ankle Int 2005;26(8):583–9.
18. Han SH, Lee JW, Lee DY, et al. Radiographic changes and clinical results of osteochondral defects of the talus with and without subchondral cysts. Foot Ankle Int 2006;27(12):1109–14.
19. Kono M, Takao M, Naito K, et al. Retrograde drilling for osteochondral lesions of the talar dome. Am J Sports Med 2006;34(9):1450–6.
20. Kumai T, Takakura Y, Higashiyama I, et al. Arthroscopic drilling for the treatment of osteochondral lesions of the talus. J Bone Joint Surg Am 1999;81(9):1229–35.
21. Robinson DE, Winson IG, Harries WJ, et al. Arthroscopic treatment of osteochondral lesions of the talus. J Bone Joint Surg Br 2003;85(7):989–93.
22. Savva N, Jabur M, Davies M, et al. Osteochondral lesions of the talus: results of repeat arthroscopic debridement. Foot Ankle Int 2007;28(6):669–73.
23. Schuman L, Struijs PA, van Dijk CN. Arthroscopic treatment for osteochondral defects of the talus. Results at follow-up at 2 to 11 years. J Bone Joint Surg Br 2002;84(3):364–8.
24. Lee KB, Bai LB, Park JG, et al. A comparison of arthroscopic and MRI findings in staging of osteochondral lesions of the talus. Knee Surg Sports Traumatol Arthrosc 2008;16(11):1047–51.

25. Taranow WS, Bisignani GA, Towers JD, et al. Retrograde drilling of osteochondral lesions of the medial talar dome. Foot Ankle Int 1999;20(8):474–80.

26. Hyer CF, Berlet GC, Philbin TM, et al. Retrograde drilling of osteochondral lesions of the talus. Foot Ankle Spec 2008;1(4):207–9.

27. Choi WJ, Park KK, Kim BS, et al. Osteochondral lesion of the talus: is there a critical defect size for poor outcome? Am J Sports Med 2009;37(10):1974–80.

28. Chuckpaiwong B, Berkson EM, Theodore GH. Microfracture for osteochondral lesions of the ankle: outcome analysis and outcome predictors of 105 cases. Arthroscopy 2008;24(1):106–12.

29. Cuttica DJ, Smith WB, Hyer CF, et al. Osteochondral lesions of the talus: predictors of clinical outcome. Foot Ankle Int 2011;32(11):1045–51.

30. Christensen JC, Driscoll HL, Tencer AF. 1994 William J. Stickel Gold Award. Contact characteristics of the ankle joint. Part 2. The effects of talar dome cartilage defects. J Am Podiatr Med Assoc 1994;84(11):537–47.

31. Deol P, Berlet GC, Hyer CF, et al. Age stratification of outcomes for osteochondral lesions of the talus. Presented at American Orthopedic Foot and Ankle Society Summer Meeting. Vancouver, July 15-18, 2009.

32. Choi WJ, Kim BS, Lee JW. Osteochondral lesion of the talus: could age be an indication for arthroscopic treatment? Am J Sports Med 2012;40(2):419–24.

33. Scranton PE Jr, McDermott JE. Treatment of type V osteochondral lesions of the talus with ipsilateral knee osteochondral autografts. Foot Ankle Int 2001;22(5):380–4.

34. Al-Shaikh RA, Chou LB, Mann JA, et al. Autologous osteochondral grafting for talar cartilage defects. Foot Ankle Int 2002;23(5):381–9.

35. Assenmacher JA, Kelikian AS, Gottlob C, et al. Arthroscopically assisted autologous osteochondral transplantation for osteochondral lesions of the talar dome: an MRI and clinical follow-up study. Foot Ankle Int 2001;22(7):544–51.

36. Hangody L, Fules P. Autologous osteochondral mosaicplasty for the treatment of full-thickness defects of weight-bearing joints: ten years of experimental and clinical experience. J Bone Joint Surg Am 2003;85(Suppl 2):25–32.

37. Kreuz PC, Steinwachs M, Erggelet C, et al. Mosaicplasty with autogenous talar autograft for osteochondral lesions of the talus after failed primary arthroscopic management: a prospective study with a 4-year follow-up. Am J Sports Med 2006;34(1):55–63.

38. Lee CH, Chao KH, Huang GS, et al. Osteochondral autografts for osteochondritis dissecans of the talus. Foot Ankle Int 2003;24(11):815–22.

39. Sammarco GJ, Makwana NK. Treatment of talar osteochondral lesions using local osteochondral graft. Foot Ankle Int 2002;23(8):693–8.

40. Gobbi A, Francisco RA, Lubowitz JH, et al. Osteochondral lesions of the talus: randomized controlled trial comparing chondroplasty, microfracture, and osteochondral autograft transplantation. Arthroscopy 2006;22(10):1085–92.

41. Hangody L, Kish G, Modis L, et al. Mosaicplasty for the treatment of osteochondritis dissecans of the talus: two to seven year results in 36 patients. Foot Ankle Int 2001;22(7):552–8.

42. Scranton PE Jr, Frey CC, Feder KS. Outcome of osteochondral autograft transplantation for type-V cystic osteochondral lesions of the talus. J Bone Joint Surg Br 2006;88(5):614–9.

43. Rama KR, Apsingi S, Poovali S, et al. Timing of tourniquet release in knee arthroplasty. Meta-analysis of randomized, controlled trials. J Bone Joint Surg Am 2007;89(4):699–705.

44. Williams SK, Amiel D, Ball ST, et al. Prolonged storage effects on the articular cartilage of fresh human osteochondral allografts. J Bone Joint Surg Am 2003;85(11):2111–20.
45. Adams SB Jr, Viens NA, Easley ME, et al. Midterm results of osteochondral lesions of the talar shoulder treated with fresh osteochondral allograft transplantation. J Bone Joint Surg Am 2011;93(7):648–54.
46. Berlet GC, Hyer CF, Philbin TM, et al. Does fresh osteochondral allograft transplantation of talar osteochondral defects improve function? Clin Orthop Relat Res 2011;469(8):2356–66.
47. El-Rashidy H, Villacis D, Omar I, et al. Fresh osteochondral allograft for the treatment of cartilage defects of the talus: a retrospective review. J Bone Joint Surg Am 2011;93(17):1634–40.
48. Gortz S, De Young AJ, Bugbee WD. Fresh osteochondral allografting for osteochondral lesions of the talus. Foot Ankle Int 2010;31(4):283–90.
49. Hahn DB, Aanstoos ME, Wilkins RM. Osteochondral lesions of the talus treated with fresh talar allografts. Foot Ankle Int 2010;31(4):277–82.
50. Raikin SM. Fresh osteochondral allografts for large-volume cystic osteochondral defects of the talus. J Bone Joint Surg Am 2009;91(12):2818–26.
51. Giannini S, Buda R, Grigolo B, et al. The detached osteochondral fragment as a source of cells for autologous chondrocyte implantation (ACI) in the ankle joint. Osteoarthritis Cartilage 2005;13(7):601–7.
52. Baums MH, Heidrich G, Schultz W, et al. Autologous chondrocyte transplantation for treating cartilage defects of the talus. J Bone Joint Surg Am 2006; 88(2):303–8.
53. Giannini S, Battaglia M, Buda R, et al. Surgical treatment of osteochondral lesions of the talus by open-field autologous chondrocyte implantation: a 10-year follow-up clinical and magnetic resonance imaging T2-mapping evaluation. Am J Sports Med 2009;37(Suppl 1):112S–8S.
54. Koulalis D, Schultz W, Heyden M. Autologous chondrocyte transplantation for osteochondritis dissecans of the talus. Clin Orthop Relat Res 2002;(395):186–92.
55. Nam EK, Ferkel RD, Applegate GR. Autologous chondrocyte implantation of the ankle: a 2- to 5-year follow-up. Am J Sports Med 2009;37(2):274–84.
56. Whittaker JP, Smith G, Makwana N, et al. Early results of autologous chondrocyte implantation in the talus. J Bone Joint Surg Br 2005;87(2):179–83.
57. Wood JJ, Malek MA, Frassica FJ, et al. Autologous cultured chondrocytes: adverse events reported to the United States Food and Drug Administration. J Bone Joint Surg Am 2006;88(3):503–7.
58. Giza E, Sullivan M, Ocel D, et al. Matrix-induced autologous chondrocyte implantation of talus articular defects. Foot Ankle Int 2010;31(9):747–53.
59. Schneider TE, Karaikudi S. Matrix-induced autologous chondrocyte implantation (MACI) grafting for osteochondral lesions of the talus. Foot Ankle Int 2009;30(9):810–4.
60. O'Driscoll SW. The healing and regeneration of articular cartilage. J Bone Joint Surg Am 1998;80(12):1795–812.
61. Koch S, Kampen WU, Laprell H. Cartilage and bone morphology in osteochondritis dissecans. Knee Surg Sports Traumatol Arthrosc 1997;5(1):42–5.
62. Uozumi H, Sugita T, Aizawa T, et al. Histologic findings and possible causes of osteochondritis dissecans of the knee. Am J Sports Med 2009;37(10):2003–8.
63. Heckman JD, Ryaby JP, McCabe J, et al. Acceleration of tibial fracture-healing by non-invasive, low-intensity pulsed ultrasound. J Bone Joint Surg Am 1994; 76(1):26–34.

64. Rubin C, Bolander M, Ryaby JP, et al. The use of low-intensity ultrasound to accelerate the healing of fractures. J Bone Joint Surg Br 2001;83(2):259–70.
65. Xavier CAM DL. Estimulaca ultra-sonica de calo osseo: applicaca clinica. Rev Brasil Ortop 1983;18:73–80 [in Portuguese].
66. Xavier CAM Duarte L. Treatment of nonunions by ultrasound stimulation: first clinical applications. Annual Meeting of The American Academy of Orthopedic Surgeons. San Francisco, January 25, 1987.
67. Xiao-lin J, Wen-zhi C, Kun Z, et al. Effects of low-intensity pulsed ultrasound in repairing injured articular cartilage. Chin J Traumatol 2005;8(3):175–8.
68. Nishikori T, Ochi M, Uchio Y, et al. Effects of low-intensity pulsed ultrasound on proliferation and chondroitin sulfate synthesis of cultured chondrocytes embedded in Atelocollagen gel. J Biomed Mater Res 2002;59(2):201–6.
69. Parvizi J, Wu CC, Lewallen DG, et al. Low-intensity ultrasound stimulates proteoglycan synthesis in rat chondrocytes by increasing aggrecan gene expression. J Orthop Res 1999;17(4):488–94.
70. Yang KH, Parvizi J, Wang SJ, et al. Exposure to low-intensity ultrasound increases aggrecan gene expression in a rat femur fracture model. J Orthop Res 1996;14(5):802–9.
71. Zhang ZJ, Huckle J, Francomano CA, et al. The influence of pulsed low-intensity ultrasound on matrix production of chondrocytes at different stages of differentiation: an explant study. Ultrasound Med Biol 2002;28(11–12):1547–53.
72. Ebisawa K, Hata K, Okada K, et al. Ultrasound enhances transforming growth factor beta-mediated chondrocyte differentiation of human mesenchymal stem cells. Tissue Eng 2004;10(5–6):921–9.
73. Leung KS, Cheung WH, Zhang C, et al. Low intensity pulsed ultrasound stimulates osteogenic activity of human periosteal cells. Clin Orthop Relat Res 2004;(418):253–9.
74. Reher P, Elbeshir el-NI, Harvey W, et al. The stimulation of bone formation in vitro by therapeutic ultrasound. Ultrasound Med Biol 1997;23(8):1251–8.
75. Brighton CT, Unger AS, Stambough JL. In vitro growth of bovine articular cartilage chondrocytes in various capacitively coupled electrical fields. J Orthop Res 1984;2(1):15–22.
76. Nogami H, Aoki H, Okagawa T, et al. Effects of electric current on chondrogenesis in vitro. Clin Orthop Relat Res 1982;(163):243–7.
77. Rodan GA, Bourret LA, Norton LA. DNA synthesis in cartilage cells is stimulated by oscillating electric fields. Science 1978;199(4329):690–2.
78. Lippiello L, Chakkalakal D, Connolly JF. Pulsing direct current-induced repair of articular cartilage in rabbit osteochondral defects. J Orthop Res 1990;8(2):266–75.
79. Bodamyali T, Bhatt B, Hughes FJ, et al. Pulsed electromagnetic fields simultaneously induce osteogenesis and upregulate transcription of bone morphogenetic proteins 2 and 4 in rat osteoblasts in vitro. Biochem Biophys Res Commun 1998;250(2):458–61.
80. Wang Z, Clark CC, Brighton CT. Up-regulation of bone morphogenetic proteins in cultured murine bone cells with use of specific electric fields. J Bone Joint Surg Am 2006;88(5):1053–65.
81. Baker B, Becker RO, Spadaro J. A study of electrochemical enhancement of articular cartilage repair. Clin Orthop Relat Res 1974;(102):251–67.
82. Baker B, Spadaro J, Marino A, et al. Electrical stimulation of articular cartilage regeneration. Ann N Y Acad Sci 1974;238:491–9.

83. Akai M, Hayashi K. Effect of electrical stimulation on musculoskeletal systems; a meta-analysis of controlled clinical trials. Bioelectromagnetics 2002;23(2):132–43.
84. Hung CT, Lima EG, Mauck RL, et al. Anatomically shaped osteochondral constructs for articular cartilage repair. J Biomech 2003;36(12):1853–64.
85. O'Loughlin PF, Heyworth BE, Kennedy JG. Current concepts in the diagnosis and treatment of osteochondral lesions of the ankle. Am J Sports Med 2010; 38(2):392–404.
86. Athanasiou KA, Shah AR, Hernandez RJ, et al. Basic science of articular cartilage repair. Clin Sports Med 2001;20(2):223–47.
87. Chen Y, Bloemen V, Impens S, et al. Characterization and optimization of cell seeding in scaffolds by factorial design: quality by design approach for skeletal tissue engineering. Tissue Eng Part C Methods 2011;17(12):1211–21.
88. Uebersax L, Hagenmuller H, Hofmann S, et al. Effect of scaffold design on bone morphology in vitro. Tissue Eng 2006;12(12):3417–29.
89. Han SH, Kim YH, Park MS, et al. Histological and biomechanical properties of regenerated articular cartilage using chondrogenic bone marrow stromal cells with a PLGA scaffold in vivo. J Biomed Mater Res Part A 2008;87(4):850–61.
90. Cuttica DJ, Shockley JA, Hyer CF, et al. Correlation of MRI edema and clinical outcomes following microfracture of osteochondral lesions of the talus. Foot Ankle Spec 2011;4(5):274–9.
91. Tytherleigh-Strong G, Hurtig M, Miniaci A. Intra-articular hyaluronan following autogenous osteochondral grafting of the knee. Arthroscopy 2005;21(8): 999–1005.
92. Bonnet CS, Walsh DA. Osteoarthritis, angiogenesis and inflammation. Rheumatology 2005;44(1):7–16.
93. Deckers MM, van Bezooijen RL, van der Horst G, et al. Bone morphogenetic proteins stimulate angiogenesis through osteoblast-derived vascular endothelial growth factor A. Endocrinology 2002;143(4):1545–53.
94. Pufe T, Petersen W, Tillmann B, et al. The splice variants VEGF121 and VEGF189 of the angiogenic peptide vascular endothelial growth factor are expressed in osteoarthritic cartilage. Arthritis Rheum 2001;44(5):1082–8.
95. Pleimann JH, Davis WH, Cohen BE, et al. Viscosupplementation for the arthritic ankle. Foot Ankle Clin 2002;7(3):489–94.
96. Divine JG, Zazulak BT, Hewett TE. Viscosupplementation for knee osteoarthritis: a systematic review. Clin Orthop Relat Res 2007;455:113–22.
97. Cohen MM, Altman RD, Hollstrom R, et al. Safety and efficacy of intra-articular sodium hyaluronate (Hyalgan) in a randomized, double-blind study for osteoarthritis of the ankle. Foot Ankle Int 2008;29(7):657–63.
98. Migliore A, Giovannangeli F, Bizzi E, et al. Viscosupplementation in the management of ankle osteoarthritis: a review. Arch Orthop Trauma Surg 2011;131(1): 139–47.
99. Sun SF, Chou YJ, Hsu CW, et al. Hyaluronic acid as a treatment for ankle osteoarthritis. Curr Rev Musculoskelet Med 2009;2(2):78–82.
100. van Dijk CN, Reilingh ML, Zengerink M, et al. Osteochondral defects in the ankle: why painful? Knee Surg Sports Traumatol Arthrosc 2010;18(5):570–80.
101. Nakamae A, Engebretsen L, Bahr R, et al. Natural history of bone bruises after acute knee injury: clinical outcome and histopathological findings. Knee Surg Sports Traumatol Arthrosc 2006;14(12):1252–8.
102. Vellet AD, Marks PH, Fowler PJ, et al. Occult posttraumatic osteochondral lesions of the knee: prevalence, classification, and short-term sequelae evaluated with MR imaging. Radiology 1991;178(1):271–6.

103. Neuhold A, Hofmann S, Engel A, et al. Bone marrow edema of the hip: MR findings after core decompression. J Comput Assist Tomogr 1992;16(6):951–5.
104. McCarthy EF, Frassica FJ. Osteonecrosis. In: Pathology of bone and joint disorders: with clinical and radiographic correlation. Philadelphia: WB Saunders; 1998. p. 135–44.
105. Tonbul M, Guzelant AY, Gonen A, et al. Relationship between the size of bone marrow edema of the talus and ankle pain. J Am Podiatr Med Assoc 2011; 101(5):430–6.
106. Hoffmann M, Petersen JP, Schroder M, et al. Accuracy analysis of a novel electromagnetic navigation procedure versus a standard fluoroscopic method for retrograde drilling of osteochondritis dissecans lesions of the knee. Am J Sports Med 2012;40(4):920–6.
107. Rosenberger RE, Bale RJ, Fink C, et al. Computer-assisted drilling of the lower extremity. Techniques and indications. Unfallchirurg 2002;105(4):353–8.
108. Rosenberger RE, Fink C, Bale RJ, et al. Computer-assisted minimally invasive treatment of osteochondrosis dissecans of the talus. Oper Orthop Traumatol 2006;18(4):300–16.
109. Aspenberg P, Van der Vis H. Migration, particles, and fluid pressure. A discussion of causes of prosthetic loosening. Clin Orthop Relat Res 1998;(352): 75–80.
110. Durr HD, Martin H, Pellengahr C, et al. The cause of subchondral bone cysts in osteoarthrosis: a finite element analysis. Acta Orthop Scand 2004;75(5):554–8.
111. Johansson L, Edlund U, Fahlgren A, et al. Bone resorption induced by fluid flow. J Biomech Eng 2009;131(9):094505.
112. Schmalzried TP, Akizuki KH, Fedenko AN, et al. The role of access of joint fluid to bone in periarticular osteolysis. A report of four cases. J Bone Joint Surg Am 1997;79(3):447–52.
113. Van der Vis HM, Aspenberg P, Marti RK, et al. Fluid pressure causes bone resorption in a rabbit model of prosthetic loosening. Clin Orthop Relat Res 1998;(350):201–8.
114. Astrand J, Skripitz R, Skoglund B, et al. A rat model for testing pharmacologic treatments of pressure-related bone loss. Clin Orthop Relat Res 2003;(409): 296–305.
115. Hunt KJ, Lee AT, Lindsey DP, et al. Osteochondral lesions of the talus: effect of defect size and plantarflexion angle on ankle joint stresses. Am J Sports Med 2012;40(4):895–901.
116. van Bergen CJ, Reilingh ML, van Dijk CN. Tertiary osteochondral defect of the talus treated by a novel contoured metal implant. Knee Surg Sports Traumatol Arthrosc 2011;19(6):999–1003.
117. van Bergen CJ, Zengerink M, Blankevoort L, et al. Novel metallic implantation technique for osteochondral defects of the medial talar dome. A cadaver study. Acta Orthop 2010;81(4):495–502.
118. Adkisson HD 4th, Martin JA, Amendola RL, et al. The potential of human allogeneic juvenile chondrocytes for restoration of articular cartilage. Am J Sports Med 2010;38(7):1324–33.
119. Zheng H, Martin JA, Duwayri Y, et al. Impact of aging on rat bone marrow-derived stem cell chondrogenesis. J Gerontol A Biol Sci Med Sci 2007;62(2): 136–48.
120. Knutsen G, Engebretsen L, Ludvigsen TC, et al. Autologous chondrocyte implantation compared with microfracture in the knee. A randomized trial. J Bone Joint Surg Am 2004;86(3):455–64.

121. Steadman JR, Briggs KK, Rodrigo JJ, et al. Outcomes of microfracture for traumatic chondral defects of the knee: average 11-year follow-up. Arthroscopy 2003;19(5):477–84.
122. Babbush CA, Kevy SV, Jacobson MS. An in vitro and in vivo evaluation of autologous platelet concentrate in oral reconstruction. Implant Dent 2003;12(1): 24–34.
123. Gandhi A, Bibbo C, Pinzur M, et al. The role of platelet-rich plasma in foot and ankle surgery. Foot Ankle Clin 2005;10(4):621–37, viii.
124. Joyce ME, Jingushi S, Scully SP, et al. Role of growth factors in fracture healing. Prog Clin Biol Res 1991;365:391–416.
125. Brehm W, Aklin B, Yamashita T, et al. Repair of superficial osteochondral defects with an autologous scaffold-free cartilage construct in a caprine model: implantation method and short-term results. Osteoarthritis Cartilage 2006;14(12): 1214–26.
126. Munirah S, Samsudin OC, Chen HC, et al. Articular cartilage restoration in load-bearing osteochondral defects by implantation of autologous chondrocyte-fibrin constructs: an experimental study in sheep. J Bone Joint Surg Br 2007;89(8): 1099–109.
127. Hiraki Y, Inoue H, Asada A, et al. Differential modulation of growth and phenotypic expression of chondrocytes in sparse and confluent cultures by growth factors in cartilage. J Bone Miner Res 1990;5(10):1077–85.
128. Rosier RN, O'Keefe RJ, Hicks DG. The potential role of transforming growth factor beta in fracture healing. Clin Orthop Relat Res 1998;(355 Suppl): S294–300.
129. Sessions CM, Emler CA, Schalch DS. Interaction of insulin-like growth factor II with rat chondrocytes: receptor binding, internalization, and degradation. Endocrinology 1987;120(5):2108–16.
130. Wang EA, Rosen V, D'Alessandro JS, et al. Recombinant human bone morphogenic protein induces bone formation. Proc Natl Acad Sci U S A 1990;87(6): 579–92.
131. Sellers RS, Peluso D, Morris EA. The effect of recombinant human bone morphogenetic protein-2 (rhBMP-2) on the healing of full-thickness defects of articular cartilage. J Bone Joint Surg Am 1997;79(10):1452–63.
132. Sellers RS, Zhang R, Glasson SS, et al. Repair of articular cartilage defects one year after treatment with recombinant human bone morphogenetic protein-2 (rhBMP-2). J Bone Joint Surg Am 2000;82(2):151–60.
133. Nejadnik H, Daldrup-Link HE. Engineering stem cells for treatment of osteochondral defects. Skeletal Radiol 2012;41(1):1–4.
134. Niemeyer P, Fechner K, Milz S, et al. Comparison of mesenchymal stem cells from bone marrow and adipose tissue for bone regeneration in a critical size defect of the sheep tibia and the influence of platelet-rich plasma. Biomaterials 2010;31(13):3572–9.
135. Rodrigues MT, Gomes ME, Reis RL. Current strategies for osteochondral regeneration: from stem cells to pre-clinical approaches. Curr Opin Biotechnol 2011; 22(5):726–33.
136. Nishimori M, Deie M, Kanaya A, et al. Repair of chronic osteochondral defects in the rat. A bone marrow-stimulating procedure enhanced by cultured allogenic bone marrow mesenchymal stromal cells. J Bone Joint Surg Br 2006;88(9):1236–44.
137. Tatebe M, Nakamura R, Kagami H, et al. Differentiation of transplanted mesenchymal stem cells in a large osteochondral defect in rabbit. Cytotherapy 2005; 7(6):520–30.

138. Wakitani S, Goto T, Pineda SJ, et al. Mesenchymal cell-based repair of large, full-thickness defects of articular cartilage. J Bone Joint Surg Am 1994;76(4): 579–92.

139. Duke J, Moore J, Montufar-Solis D. Continuing studies of "cells" flight hardware. Physiologist 1989;32(1 Suppl):S57–8.

140. Duke PJ, Arizpe J, Montufar-Solis D. Cartilage formation in the cells "double bubble" hardware. Physiologist 1991;34(1 Suppl):S76–7.

141. Duke PJ, Daane EL, Montufar-Solis D. Studies of chondrogenesis in rotating systems. J Cell Biochem 1993;51(3):274–82.

142. Goodwin TJ, Jessup JM, Wolf DA. Morphologic differentiation of colon carcinoma cell lines HT-29 and HT-29KM in rotating-wall vessels. In Vitro Cell Dev Biol 1992;28A(1):47–60.

143. Tsao YD, Goodwin TJ, Wolf DA, et al. Responses of gravity level variations on the NASA/JSC bioreactor system. Physiologist 1992;35(1 Suppl):S49–50.

144. Veldhuijzen JP, Huisman AH, Vermedien JP, et al. The growth of cartilage cells in vitro and the effects of intermittent compressive forces: a histological evaluation. Connect Tissue Res 1987;16:187–96.

Talus Osteochondral Bruises and Defects: Diagnosis and Differentiation

Graham A. McCollum, FCS Orth(SA), MMED(UCT)[a,b],
James D.F. Calder, TD, MD, FRCS(Tr&Orth), FFSEM(UK)[a,b],*,
Umile Giuseppe Longo, MD, MS[c], Mattia Loppini, MD[c],
Giovanni Romeo, MD[c], C. Niek van Dijk, MD, PhD[d],
Nicola Maffulli, MD, MS, PhD, FRCS(Orth)[e], Vincenzo Denaro, MD[a,b]

KEYWORDS

- Bone bruise • Ankle • Talus • Osteochondral defect • Ankle sprain • Ligament tear

KEY POINTS

- Osteochondral defects (OCDs) can exist with or without associated bone bruises, but defects in the subchondral bone plate or the cartilage are present. In most cases, the lesion is posttraumatic after an ankle sprain.
- Bone bruising is shown by increased signal on T2-weighted images and decreased signal on T1-weighted images.
- Bone bruising can be evident on magnetic resonance imaging for 10 to 12 months.
- Talar bone bruises occur in up to 40% of ankle sprains.
- Ankles with OCDs and significant bruising close to the articular surface should remain nonweight bearing for 4 to 6 weeks, allowing healing of the subchondral bone plate.

INTRODUCTION

Talar bone bruising and osteochondral defects (OCDs) are increasingly being recognized after ankle trauma. The increased use of magnetic resonance imaging (MRI) is identifying lesions that may not previously have been suspected. Bone bruising of the knee after trauma and anterior cruciate ligament (ACL) injury has been extensively

[a] Chelsea & Westminster Hospital, 369 Fulham Road, London SW10 9NH, UK; [b] Fortius Clinic, 17 Fitzhardinge Street, London W1H 6EQ, UK; [c] Department of Orthopaedic and Trauma Surgery, Campus Bio-Medico University, Via Alvaro del Portillo, 200, Trigoria 00128, Rome, Italy; [d] Department of Orthopaedic Surgery, Academic Medical Center, University of Amsterdam, PO Box 22700, Amsterdam 1100 DE, The Netherlands; [e] Centre for Sports and Exercise Medicine, Barts and The London School of Medicine and Dentistry, Mile End Hospital, 275 Bancroft Road, London E1 4DG, England
* Corresponding author. Department of Orthopaedic Surgery, The University of Cape Town, Groote Schuur Hospital Observatory, Cape Town 7925, South Africa.
E-mail address: james.calder@imperial.ac.uk

Foot Ankle Clin N Am 18 (2013) 35–47
http://dx.doi.org/10.1016/j.fcl.2012.12.002
foot.theclinics.com

documented, but there is a paucity of literature regarding bone bruising in the ankle. This article reviews the available literature and concentrates on the diagnosis, prognosis, and management of posttraumatic ankle bone bruising and on differentiating the lesion from an OCD of the talus. Treatment focuses on bone bruising and the acute posttraumatic OCD.

OCD and bone bruising are distinguished by the presence or absence of a break in the subchondral bone plate.[1] Most OCDs are surrounded by bone edema and contusion in the acute setting, which can look like a bone bruise except for the presence of a subchondral bone plate injury and possible cartilage disruption. Chronic cystic OCD's may have significant associated edema in symptomatic patients. The prognosis of acute bone bruises and OCD is generally good, with most lesions healing or resolving.[2] Osteoarthritis secondary to an OCD is rare, but some lesions continue to be symptomatic and cause ankle dysfunction. Bone bruises seem to be benign, with radiologic resolution in 6 to 12 months.[3] The initial treatment of bone bruising and acute OCD is nonoperative. Surgery is reserved for symptomatic OCDs or when ligament reconstruction is performed, in which case, arthroscopic assessment is indicated, with possible debridement and microfracture of the OCD.

DEFINITION

A bone bruise is a subchondral osseous fracture of the cancellous microarchitecture with accompanied local hemorrhage and edema.[4] Minck and Deutsch[5] first described bone bruising in the knee as a distinct lesion based on MRI findings. Bone bruises are characterized by increased signal on T2-weighted images and decreased signal on T1-weighted images. The subchondral bone plate and cartilage layer above the lesion remain intact. This finding was confirmed by arthroscopy after MRI in 2 patients in this study: there was no corresponding cartilage lesion or macroscopic disruption over a confirmed bone bruise.

The bone trabecular microarchitecture fails under axial load, and a compression fracture occurs. When the overlying cartilage or the subchondral bone plate lose continuity or are disrupted, it is termed an OCD or osteochondral fracture. The differentiation is important because the prognosis and treatment may be different.

If the subchondral bone plate is broken, then the subchondral bone is exposed to the high hydrostatic pressures generated within the ankle and the surrounding hyaline cartilage, forcing fluid into the bone.[6] Synovial fluid under compression is osteolytic, and if the subchondral bone plate does not heal, a cystic OCD may develop, which can be symptomatic, progressive, and require surgical treatment.

There is a spectrum of trauma to the cartilage and subchondral bone. With increasing axial load, the initial bone bruise progresses to disruption of the cartilage and subchondral bone plate. The disease changes from a bone bruise to an OCD.

INCIDENCE

The ankle is one of the most frequently injured joints in sporting activities and in the general population.[7,8] 25–30% of people sustaining an ankle sprain have chronic pain and dysfunction, resulting in further investigation.[9] This situation may be as a result of ligament incompetence, impingement, and chondral or bony defects. Repeated trauma and instability increase the incidence of chronic pain, bone, and chondral disease.

Most injuries are inversion mechanisms, with a sprain or disruption of the lateral ligament complex. Isolated injury to the deltoid ligament is rare; it is usually associated with other significant bone, chondral, and soft tissue trauma, such as a syndesmotic injury. High ankle sprains or syndesmotic injuries account for 1% to 20%[10,11] of ankle sprains and often lead to long-term dysfunction and pain. Associated chondral and bony injuries are common. Brown and colleagues[12] identified a 78% incidence of bone bruising in the presence of a syndesmotic injury and an incidence of 11% in isolated lateral ligament tears. Deltoid injuries were associated with bone bruises in 9 of 13 (70%) cases in a review of 109 ankle ligament injuries.[13]

The incidence of bone bruises after inversion trauma with isolated injury to the lateral ligaments ranges from 7.4%[14] to 40%.[15,16] The severity of injury seems to correlate with the incidence and number of bone bruises to the talus: Pinar and colleagues[16] differentiated the grade of lateral ligament injury and compared the incidence of bone bruising. They found an incidence of 16% in isolated anterior talofibular ligament (ATFL) injuries and 50% in cases of combined ATFL and calcaneofibular (CFL), grade III injuries. The incidence of bone bruising in the knee after complete ACL rupture is high. Fowler and colleagues[17] reported an incidence of 71% to 85% in their series, and it is higher in complex multiligamentous knee injuries.[18]

CAUSE AND PATTERN

Most bone bruises and osteochondral lesions are the result of trauma. There is a small subset of OCD (medial lesions) that may not be trauma related.[19] They result from local ischemia and underlying necrosis, the cause of which is not clear but it may be hereditary, because there is a high incidence in monozygotic twins and it is bilateral in 10% of cases.[20,21]

Ankle sprains are the usual mechanism of injury, particularly in the sportsperson, but ankle fractures and high impact loading are also associated with chondral and subchondral bony injury. The most common ankle sprain is an inversion, adduction mechanism. The ATFL, then the CFL, and (rarely) the posterior talofibular (PTFL) ligaments are injured sequentially, with increasing severity of sprain.

Nishimura and colleagues[22] identified 4 patterns of bone bruising on MRI and compared the associated ligament injuries with each: (1) posterolateral talar dome, (2) posteromedial talar dome together with the medial malleolus, (3) anteromedial talus, and (4) a combination of posteromedial and anteromedial bruises. The posterolateral talar dome bruise was associated with an isolated partial ATFL tear. Posteromedial and medial malleolar bruises were sustained after inversion with the foot plantarflexed. They were associated with complete ATFL tears and an intact CFL. Anteromedial bruises were associated with dorsiflexion injuries and inversion and complete tears of the ATFL and CFL. In the fourth group, the mechanism was a combination of inversion in plantarflexion and then dorsiflexion sequentially. The clinical implication of this study is that ligament injury patterns may be identified and confirmed by the bone bruising patterns. The most common sites for OCD are anterolateral and posteromedial, with the lateral lesions being shallow and oval from the sheer force and the medial lesions deep and cup-shaped from the axial compression.[23]

Sijbrandij and colleagues[24,25] identified a 10% incidence of kissing lesions involving the talus and tibial plafond in 146 MRI scans of sequentially injured ankles. Most of these lesions were located on the posteromedial talar dome opposite the corresponding tibial bruise (Fig. 1). This situation is analogous to the kissing lesions seen in the knee.[2] Direct nonpenetrating knee trauma such as a direct blow to the patella or femoral condyle can cause a local bone bruise, separate to the typical axial load subchondral lesion.[17] Similarly, direct trauma to the medial or lateral malleoli may also cause local bone bruising. Ligament insertion avulsion can lead to local bone bruising. Traction on the underlying bone and periosteum can cause local contusions and

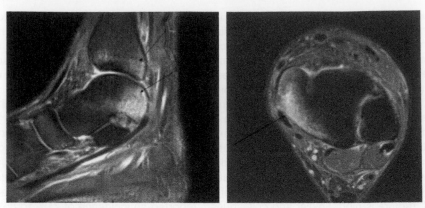

Fig. 1. Posteromedial talar bruise with corresponding tibial bruise: kissing lesion. Arrows show increased signal intensity on the T2 weighted image.

positive MRI findings. They occur at the insertion of the ATFL and CFL on the fibula and calcaneus, respectively, and the deltoid ligament insertion on the medial malleolus.[22]

CLINICAL PRESENTATION AND EXAMINATION

As mentioned earlier, ankle injuries are common. It is estimated that there is 1 ankle inversion injury per 10 000 persons per day.[26] Of these, injuries 25% to 30% have residual symptoms, for a variety of reasons. One reason may be an OCD or a bone bruise. After ankle trauma, patients typically experience pain from the soft tissue and ligament injury, lasting 4 to 6 weeks. If significant pain, stiffness, and swelling are still a feature after this time, an OCD should be suspected. Locking, clicking, or catching are symptoms of a displaced fragment. Taga and colleagues[27] performed an arthroscopy before ligament stabilization in 31 patients complaining of ongoing pain after an ankle sprain. These investigators found chondral injuries in 89% of acute injuries (6–8 weeks) and 95% of chronic (>3 months) injuries. Van Dijk and colleagues[28] identified 20 acute cartilage injuries out of 30 ankles undergoing arthroscopy before ligament stabilization. These investigators reported the high incidence of cartilage injury (19 of 20) to the medial malleolus and the opposite medial facet of the talus. They correlated the incidence of cartilage injury with higher-velocity injury and impact sports such as jumping or landing from a height.

Not all cartilage lesions are visible on MRI. Takao and colleagues[29] identified a 27% incidence of cartilage injury at arthroscopy not evident on MRI. There was no evidence of bone bruising, despite arthroscopically proven cartilage defects in this group. These studies show that sometimes arthroscopy is an important diagnostic and therapeutic tool in the chronically painful ankle after a sprain.

Repeated injury may be a cause of persistent bone bruising and OCD propagation. Chronic ankle instability places the subchondral bone and cartilage under significant repetitive load, delaying edema resorption and healing of subchondral microfracture.[29] Hindfoot or tibial malalignment may perpetuate chronic ankle instability and focal load on the injured ankle cartilage and subchondral bone. This malalignment needs to be examined for in all cases.

Generally, OCDs do not result in synovitis or a large joint effusion unless there is a loose body, a large defect, or a displaced fragment, in which case, synovitis can be a feature, together with symptoms of locking, clicking, stiffness, and swelling. The associated deep ankle pain is difficult to localize and is worse during and after exercise.[30] A large displaced OCD may be associated with palpable synovitis and direct talar pain on deep palpation if the lesion is anterior on the talus.[29] Bone bruising does not usually result in synovitis and pain is not common: if pain is experienced, it is deep ankle pain, worse during and after loading or exercise. Cartilage is not innervated and is not the source of pain. The subchondral bone is innervated, with both unmyelinated and myelinated fibers within the Haversian system. Mach and colleagues[31] reported that the greatest concentration of these nerve fibers and nocireceptors occur in the proximal and distal ends of mouse femur bones, particularly in the subchondral area. Pain probably arises because of an increase in intraosseous pressure, and macrophage-mediated acidosis of the microenvironment, which excites the high concentration of nerves.

INVESTIGATION

Radiographs are important. They do not show bone bruising but may reveal large osteochondral lesions and associated fractures. Avulsion fractures of the ATFL, CFL, or deltoid may be evident and indicate significant ligamentous injury. Hindfoot and tibial alignment can be assessed on radiographs. Ankle injury severity correlates with the incidence and degree of bone bruising and OCD.[16] Therefore, ligamentous injury evident on radiographs may lead to suspicion of an osseous or chondral injury or both.

MRI is the investigation of choice to identify, quantify, and differentiate chondral and osseous bruising. Visualization and detection of injury to the medial, lateral, and syndesmotic ligaments is possible at the same time. A bone bruise appears as an ill-defined semicircular area of abnormal signal intensity in the subchondral bone. The signal intensity is increased on T2-weighted images, reflecting intraosseous edema and hemorrhage. T1 images appear hypointense, reflecting the anatomic disruption of the normal microarchitecture. Fat-saturated or short tau inversion recovery sequences are accurate at detecting osseous edema and hemorrhage.[5,32] An OCD or fracture is differentiated by the disruption of the subchondral bone plate. This disruption is visualized as a low-intensity line extending through the plate to the undersurface of the cartilage.[33] Griffith and colleagues[34] showed the accuracy of 3.0-Tesler high-resolution MR in visualizing the articular surface, the subchondral bone plate and surrounding bone edema noting it to be superior to lower-field 1.5-T scans and suggested that it be used with all suspected OCD and bone bruises. Computed tomography (CT) scanning may be helpful in visualizing the precise anatomy and behavior of larger cystic and displaced lesions.

CLASSIFICATION

Roemer and Bohndorf[35] provided an MRI classification of bone bruising based on their knee research: stage 1, bone edema only; stage 2, bone edema and spongious impaction; stage 3, associated with microfracture, progressing to osteochondral fracture through the subchondral bone plate. This classification shows the continuum of injury, progressing with increasing severity from a simple contusion to a fracture of the cartilage and underlying bone. Essentially, stage 3 in this classification is an OCD. The most commonly used radiograph-based classification of OCD is that of Berndt and Harty.[36] Stage 1 is a compressed cartilage segment, stage 2 an avulsed but attached segment, stage 3 is a completely detached but minimally displaced fragment, and stage 4 is a loose, displaced fragment. Numerous CT, MRI, and arthroscopic classifications exist. They all originate from the original Berndt and Harty[36] classification, with modifications showing the increasing instability and displacement of the lesion.[37,38]

PROGNOSIS

Athletes and professional sportspeople are increasingly obtaining MRI scans shortly after ankle trauma, identifying chondral and bony injury amongst other soft tissue damage. It is important to be able to predict which injuries or severities lead to chronic ankle problems or dysfunction and intervene surgically or nonsurgically to improve outcome and hasten recovery. To achieve this goal, an understanding is needed of the natural history of bone bruises and OCD. Generally, the prognosis of bone bruising is good. It has been learnt from the knee that bone bruising after ACL trauma is common and that most of these knees do not suffer significant chondral loss as a result of the underlying contusion. This finding is true if the subchondral plate is intact and there is no significant cartilage loss or fracture.[39] Typically, the tibial and femoral bruises resolve by 4 to 6 weeks on serial MRI scans, healing from the periphery to the center.[5] Vellet and colleagues[15] showed that 67% of knees sustaining geographic or linear lesions involving the subchondral bone plate had evidence of osteochondral sequelae compared with a 100% resolution of reticular lesions distant from the joint surface at 6 to 8 weeks. Resolution of ankle bone bruising is slower. Sijbrandij and colleagues[24] showed the persistence of edema in the talus for 11 to 12 months on average and up to 17 months after contusion with repeat MRI scans. There was clinical improvement in symptoms long before the MRI resolution.

Alanen and colleagues[40] prospectively studied a series of 95 inversion ankle injuries. They identified an incidence of bone bruising of 27%. The presence of a bone bruise made no difference to the time to return to work, walking, or physical activity at 3 months after injury. Zanetti and colleagues[41] followed 29 ankle injuries with early postinjury MRI and an MRI at 3 months. Six patients had bone bruises identified on the first MRI. All these bruises persisted at the 3-month follow-up MRI scan, but their outcome was not significantly different from patients with similar ligament injuries without bone bruises. These investigators' conclusion was that the degree of ligament injury determines the clinical outcome, not the presence of a bone bruise. Few bone bruises are symptomatic and they are often an incidental finding.[42] The degree of bone bruising and number of bruises has been shown to correlate with degree of ligament disruption.[4]

When the bone bruise is continuous with the ankle joint (a disrupted subchondral bone plate and termed an OCD), spontaneous healing is less predictable, because of joint and cartilage fluid being forced into the fissure with each loading cycle.[43] When a distinct fragment is present, synovial fluid surrounds it and prevents bone healing. The high intraosseous pressure and valve effect of the overlying remaining cartilage can lead to cyst formation and contribute to pain. Cyst formation leads to unsupported cartilage, which can degenerate in response, exposing the underlying subchondral bone.[44] Healing of the subchondral bone plate is critical to arrest the progression of an OCD if detected early.

MANAGEMENT

There is little high-level evidence to guide the early management of bone bruises. As mentioned earlier, the natural history of bone bruises is benign, but the integrity of the subchondral bone plate is critical to the resolution or possible propagation to an OCD. High-resolution MRI has the ability to accurately show the cartilage and underlying bone plate. If significant edema occurs adjacent to the plate or if the plate is shown to be broken, the presence of a communication of the subchondral bone with the joint and cartilage must be suspected. This finding may change treatment strategies.

Bone bruises and osteochondral injuries are associated with ligament tears in most cases, and treatment depends on the level of athlete and the degree of tear. Most lateral ligament sprains are grade 1 or 2. The accepted treatment of these injuries is nonsurgical, consisting of a short period (5–7days) of immobilization and nonweight bearing in a cast or boot followed by functional rehabilitation. This rehabilitation entails increasing weight bearing, proprioception training, and strengthening.[45] The treatment of grade 3 tears is controversial. A Cochrane review[46] suggested that functional rehabilitation was superior to surgery, with fewer complications and stiffness, but there was an increased laxity and instability in conservatively treated patients. For this reason, there is a trend to treat the professional athlete surgically with ligament repair, although high-level evidence is lacking. Arthroscopy at the time of the ligament repair allows assessment of the articular surface, removal of loose bodies, and debridement of chondral injuries if necessary. Cartilage-stimulating restorative procedures are reserved for chronic symptomatic lesions or large primary areas of cartilage loss.

Repeat chondral injury from incompetent lateral ligaments results in poor healing of a bone bruise and propagation of an OCD. If identified as a cause of the disease, ligaments should be repaired or reconstructed after careful assessment of hindfoot and ankle alignment.

Weight bearing has been shown to substantially increase the hydrostatic pressure in the congruent ankle joint. This pressure is greatest over the shoulders of the talus.[47] Whether surgical or nonsurgical treatment is chosen to treat the ligament tear, the bone bruise or OCD should be carefully evaluated. If a break in the cartilage or the subchondral bone plate is seen on early MRI, a period of nonweight bearing should be instigated. The period is difficult to determine because it is not known how long the bone plate takes to heal. Some investigators have suggested 2 to 4 weeks,[24,41] whereas others[48] have suggested longer periods of up to 6 weeks for proven posttraumatic OCD. Prolonged non-weight bearing and immobilization in a cast or boot leads to muscle atrophy and stiffness, and therefore physical therapy should be continued through this period to maintain range of motion and strength.

Bone bruises that are not located near the articular surface may be treated less aggressively. Weight bearing can begin as permitted in the post lateral ligament rehabilitation protocol. Alanen and colleagues[40] showed no difference in the outcome of patients with bone bruises who followed the functional rehabilitation protocol compared with patients without bone bruises. If rehabilitation progress is slow, the patient should be reassessed and a repeat MRI performed.

Although bone bruises are benign, the propagation to a symptomatic OCD is concerning and may be altered by other nonsurgical intervention. Alternative nonsurgical therapies have been researched; perhaps, these have a role to play in achieving bone and cartilage healing, arresting progression, and aiding resolution of a bone bruise with subchondral plate disruption.

Shock wave therapy is commonly used for the treatment of soft tissue conditions and some evidence suggests there are beneficial effects on bone and cartilage.[49,50] High-energy treatment requires some form of general anesthesia or sedation, but low-energy treatment can be performed in the office with no anesthesia required. The same amount of energy flux density can be dissipated to the tissue by increasing the pulse cycles of the low-energy treatment.[51] There is no evidence to suggest that the benefits of the 2 are any different for the treatment of bone and cartilage conditions.[52] The energy has both direct and indirect effects on the tissue. The shock wave creates a tensile force and cavitation bubbles after the passage of the wave.

These bubbles expand, then collapse and collide into each other, dissipating the energy. The resulting energy transfer causes a biological response: the indirect effect.

The most important effects on bone are angiogenesis, neovascularity, growth factor release, and osteogenic stem cell recruitment and differentiation.[53] Animal studies have shown the upregulation of growth factors (vascular endothelial growth factor and nitric oxidase release[54]) and increases in the production of bone morphogenic protein 2.[55] New subperiosteal bone formation and increased density and strength of treated rabbit femora have been shown.[55,56] Single-photon emission CT (SPECT) scanning after shock wave therapy has shown increased biological activity with increased absorption of technetium-labeled MDP and cortical thickening in rat tibias.[53] Wang and colleagues[57] have shown the beneficial effects and improved response to microfracture with increased fibrocartilage formation in a rabbit model and improved healing of osteochondritis dissecans of the rabbit knee. Although many of these effects have not been shown in vivo in human trials, the beneficial effects should be a source of further research because this may be a cost-effective treatment with a low risk of complications or adverse effects. We have no experience with this treatment of bone bruises or OCDs of the talus, but ongoing research may show benefit.

Platelet-rich plasma (PRP) is a delivery vehicle for bioactive proteins and growth factors essential for repair and anabolic processes in cartilage and other tissues. They include insulin-like growth factor I, platelet-derived growth factor, and transforming growth factor β1.[58] There also seems to be a role in slowing degeneration with inhibition of metalloproteinases by naturally found endoproteinase inhibitors in PRP, and PRP has been found to increase the secretion of hyaluronic acid from the synovial cells.[59] There also seems to be an antiinflammatory effect.[59]

The patient's own blood is spun in a centrifuge, removing the white and red cells retaining the factors mentioned earlier and platelets in concentrations 2 to 3 times higher than in normal blood.[60] Use of PRP is becoming more widespread and early data from studies are encouraging. The treatment of osteoarthritis of the knee is well described, with good short-term results improving pain and joint function.[61] The anabolic effects on chondrocytes have been described and they may be beneficial in the treatment of chondral or subchondral disease.[62] Mei Dan and colleagues[60] compared the intra-articular use of PRP with that of hyaluronic acid for the treatment of talar OCDs, finding statistically higher ankle scores at medium-term and short-term follow-up in the PRP treatment group. The long-term clinical effects are not known. This finding does not necessarily translate to better cartilage tissue quality, so the beneficial effects may be multifactorial, including a strong antiinflammatory component. Serra and colleagues[63] showed that PRP did not improve the biological quality of repair of OCDs in a rabbit model after microfracture and that fibrocartilage content as well as the mechanical properties were equal to a placebo group.

Several preparation protocols from different companies exist, resulting in a variety of concentrations and content of the centrifuged serum. Some require a coagulant and others a certain percentage of leukocytes and other catalysts. The duration and cycles of centrifuge vary, resulting in heterogeneous content. This situation may have significant biological implications. A certain quantity of platelets is necessary and beneficial, but too great a concentration can be inhibitory.[64] For these reasons, the treating surgeon must be familiar with a certain product and the results obtained from their specific research.[65] We have no experience with the use of PRP for the treatment of bone bruising and possible early OCD. PRP may be a good tool for the treatment of these lesions, because the complication rate is low and the intervention aims to heal the subchondral bone plate and the overlying cartilage. PRP may be indicated for significant bone bruising adjacent to the subchondral plate, but this is speculative at this point. Bone bruising distant to the subchondral plate is benign, and there is no role for the use of biological stimulation.

Conventional CT has little role in diagnosing bone bruising and is not a first-line investigation. It may reveal trabecular fractures or cortical disruptions, raising the suspicion of significant bony trauma. Dual- energy CT with calcium-eliminating techniques can show bone bruising and edema and was shown to compare well with MRI in diagnosing bruises after knee trauma in a recent study.[66] MRI remains the gold standard in diagnosing bone bruising, but significant trauma adjacent to the articular surface should raise the suspicion of a subchondral fracture; CT scanning may better visualize the bony anatomy. SPECT is a valuable diagnostic tool for imaging bone edema, osteoblastic activity, and the subchondral bone plate. Leuman and colleagues[67] showed that SPECT had better interobserver correlation in diagnosing disruption of the subchondral bone plate than MRI. Bone edema on MRI did not always correlate with increased osteoblastic activity on SPECT, showing that MRI may overestimate the size and extent of a lesion. These investigators suggested MRI and SPECT for better surgical planning in cases of early or chronic OCDs. High-definition MRI using a 3-T magnet shows the subchondral bone and plate better than lower-resolution scans, identifying and delineating fractures and OCDs.[34] CT scanning is beneficial in established OCDs, better showing the bony anatomy beneath the defect in the cartilage or the formation of an early cyst.

Serial MRI scans are indicated for those patients who remain symptomatic with deep ankle pain 6 to 8 weeks after a sprain. These scans are not indicated in confirmed cases of bone bruising because the prognosis is benign and evidence of a bruise is usually present for 6 to 12 months[24] in asymptomatic patients. If significant symptoms of deep ankle pain after bone bruise persist for 8 weeks, repeat MRI is indicated, looking for progression of the bone bruise to an OCD. In cases in which no primary MRI was performed at the time of injury, MRI should be performed at 2 to 3 months after injury if deep ankle pain persists after careful examination to exclude instability or associated soft tissue injury. There is no evidence in the foot and ankle literature of the incidence of propagation from a talar bone bruise to an OCD. The knee literature shows that bone bruising is benign and the incidence of deterioration to an OCD is rare.[1]

Return to sports and training is dependent on the soft tissue injury and degree of articular injury. Patients with grade 1 to 2 lateral ligament injuries should be permitted to train after a 6-week period of structured rehabilitation.[49] An occult benign bone bruise should not lengthen this period. An OCD lengthens the period to 10 to 12 weeks because a period of nonweight bearing of 2 to 4 weeks is indicated. Running should be restricted for at least 10 weeks to avoid displacement or disruption of a healing OCD. Grade 3 ligament injuries with an associated OCD need a longer period of rehabilitation, at least 12 weeks, or longer if the OCD requires arthroscopic cartilage debridement and bone marrow stimulation techniques. Bone bruising distant to the articular surface or when the integrity of the subchondral bone plate has been confirmed by high-resolution MRI should not limit rehabilitation and early return to activity. Caution should be exercised when significant bruising occurs close to the subchondral bone, because small breaks in the plate may be present and not visible on MRI or CT. A period of nonweight bearing (2 weeks) together with slower return to rehabilitation and sports should be instigated.

SUMMARY

Acute bone bruises of the talus after ankle injury are common. They need to be differentiated from OCDs because their management is different. Bone bruises have a benign course, with clinical resolution in 6 to 8 weeks, but MRI may show persistent edema for 6 to 12 months. The presence of a bone bruise should not delay rehabilitation unless symptoms persist or significant edema is close to the subchondral plate. Most do not cause ankle dysfunction. OCDs are essentially a fracture of the cartilage and underlying subchondral bone plate. They have a less predictable prognosis, and rehabilitation should aim at promoting healing of the fracture to avoid long-term symptoms, complications, and propagation of the lesion. A period of nonweight bearing, maintaining strength and range of motion, reduces the cyclical pressure load through the fissure and promotes healing. Surgery should be reserved for chronic symptomatic lesions (3 months after injury) or for those patients undergoing lateral ligament reconstruction in whom arthroscopic assessment is indicated.

REFERENCES

1. Rosen MA, Jackson DW, Berger PE. Occult osseous lesions documented by MRI associated with anterior cruciate ligament ruptures. Arthroscopy 1991;7:45–51.
2. Schuman L, Struijs PA, van Dijk CN. Arthroscopic treatment for osteochondral defects of the talus. Results at follow-up at 2 to 11 years. J Bone Joint Surg Br 2002;84:364–8.
3. Boks SS, Vroegindeweij D, Koes BW, et al. Follow-up of occult bone lesions detected at MR imaging: systematic review. Radiology 2006;238:853–62.
4. Yao I, Lee JK. Occult intraosseous fracture: detection with MR imaging. Radiology 1988;167:749–51.
5. Mink JH, Deutsch AL. Occult cartilage and bone injuries of the knee: detection, classification, and assessment with MR imaging. Radiology 1989;170:823–9.
6. Van Dijk CN, Reilingh ML, Zengerinck M. Osteochondral defects of the ankle: painful, why? Knee Surg Sports Traumatol Arthrosc 2010;18:570–80.
7. van Dijk CN, Molenaar AH, Cohen RH, et al. Value of arthrography after supination trauma of the ankle. Skeletal Radiol 1998;27:256–61.
8. van Dijk CN, Lim LS, Bossuyt PM, et al. Physical examination is sufficient for the diagnosis of sprained ankles. J Bone Joint Surg Br 1996;78:958–62.
9. Rijke AM, Goitz HT, McCue FC, et al. Magnetic resonance imaging of injury to the lateral ankle ligaments. Am J Sports Med 1993;21:528–34.
10. Gerber JP, Milliams GN, Scoville CR, et al. Persistent disability associated with ankle sprains; a prospective examination of an athletic population. Foot Ankle Int 1998;19:653–60.
11. Hopkinson WJ, St Pierre P, Ryan JB, et al. Syndesmosis sprains of the ankle. Foot Ankle Int 1990;10:325–30.
12. Brown KW, Morrison WB, Schweitzer ME, et al. MRI findings associated with distal tibiofibular syndesmosis injury. AJR Am J Roentgenol 2004;182:131–6.
13. Labovitz JM, Schweitzer ME. Occult osseous injuries after ankle sprains: incidence, location, pattern, and age. Foot Ankle Int 1998;19:661–7.
14. Yammine K, Fathi Y. Ankle "sprains" during sport activities with normal radiographs: incidence of associated bone and tendon injuries on MRI findings and its clinical impact. Foot (Edinb) 2011;21:176–8.
15. Vellet AD, Marks PH, Fowler PJ, et al. Occult posttraumatic osteochondral lesions of the knee: prevalence, classification, and short-term sequelae evaluated with MR imaging. Radiology 1991;178:271–6.
16. Pinar H, Akseki D, Kovanlikaya I, et al. Bone bruises detected by magnetic resonance imaging following lateral ankle sprains. Knee Surg Sports Traumatol Arthrosc 1997;5:113–7.

17. Fowler PJ. Bone injuries associated with anterior cruciate disruption. Arthroscopy 1994;10:453–69.
18. Graf BK, Cook DA, De Smet AA, et al. 'Bone bruises' on magnetic resonance imaging evaluation of anterior cruciate ligament injuries. Am J Sports Med 1993;21:220–3.
19. Ferkel RD, Scranton PE Jr. Arthroscopy of the ankle and foot. J Bone Joint Surg Am 1993;75:1233–42.
20. Woods K, Harris I. Osteochondritis dissecans of the talus in identical twins. J Bone Joint Surg Br 1995;77B:331.
21. Erban WK, Kolberg K. Simultaneous mirror image osteochondrosis dissecans in identical twins. Rofo 1981;135:357.
22. Nishimura G, Yamato M, Togawa M. Trabecular trauma of the talus and medial malleolus concurrent with lateral collateral ligamentous injuries of the ankle: evaluation with MR imaging. Skeletal Radiol 1996;25:49–54.
23. Canale ST, Belding RH. Osteochondral lesions of the talus. J Bone Joint Surg Am 1980;62:97–102.
24. Sijbrandij ES, van Gils AP, Louwerens JW, et al. Posttraumatic subchondral bone contusions and fractures of the talotibial joint: occurrence of "kissing" lesions. AJR Am J Roentgenol 2000;175:1707–10.
25. Terzidis IP, Christodoulou AG, Ploumis AL, et al. The appearance of kissing contusions in the acutely injured knee in athletes. Br J Sports Med 2004;38(5):592–6.
26. Katcherian D. Soft-tissue injuries of the ankle. In: Lutter LD, Mizel MS, Pfeffer GB, editors. Orthopaedic update knowledge. Foot and Ankle. Rosemont (IL): The American Academy of Orthopaedic Surgeons; 1994. p. 241–55.
27. Taga I, Shino K, Inoue M, et al. Articular cartilage lesions in ankles with lateral ligament injury. An arthroscopic study. Am J Sports Med 1993;21:120–6.
28. van Dijk CN, Bossuyt PM, Marti RK. Medial ankle pain after lateral ligament rupture. J Bone Joint Surg Br 1996;78:562–7.
29. Takao M, Uchio Y, Naito K, et al. Arthroscopic assessment for intra-articular disorders in residual ankle disability after sprain. Am J Sports Med 2005;33(5):686–92.
30. Ferkel RD, Zanotti RM, Komenda GA, et al. Arthroscopic treatment of chronic osteochondral lesions of the talus: long-term results. Am J Sports Med 2008; 36:1750–62.
31. Mach DB, Rogers SD, Sabino MC, et al. Origins of skeletal pain; sensory and sympathetic innervations of the mouse femur. Neuroscience 2002;113:155–66.
32. Dienst M, Blauth M. Bone bruise of the calcaneus. A case report. Clin Orthop Relat Res 2000;(378):202–5.
33. Langer I, Matthias F, Kuehn JP, et al. Acute inversion injury of the ankle without radiological abnormalities: assessment with high-field MR imaging and correlation of findings with clinical outcome. Skeletal Radiol 2011;40:423–30.
34. Griffith JF, Lau DT, Yeung DK, et al. High-resolution MR imaging of talar osteochondral lesions with new classification. Skelet Radiol 2012;41:387–99.
35. Roemer FW, Bohndorf K. Long-term osseous sequelae after acute trauma of the knee joint evaluated by MRI. Skeletal Radiol 2002;31:615–23.
36. Berndt AL, Harty M. Transchondral fractures (osteochondritis dissecans) of the talus. J Bone Joint Surg Am 1959;41:988–1020.
37. Ferkel RD, Flannigan BD, Elkins BS. MRI of the foot and ankle. Correlation of the normal anatomy with pathological conditions. Foot Ankle 1991;11(5):289–305.
38. Mint DN, Tasjian GS, Connell DA, et al. Osteochondral lesions of the talus: a new magnetic resonance imaging classification with arthroscopic correlation. Arthroscopy 2003;19(4):353–9.

39. Davies NH, Niall D, King LJ, et al. Magnetic resonance imaging of bone bruising in the acutely injured knee–short-term outcome. Clin Radiol 2004;59:439–45.
40. Alanen V, Taimela S, Kinnunen J, et al. Incidence and clinical significance of bone bruises after supination injury of the ankle. A double-blind, prospective study. J Bone Joint Surg Br 1998;80:513–5.
41. Zanetti M, De Simoni C, Wetz HH, et al. Magnetic resonance imaging of injuries to the ankle joint: can it predict clinical outcome? Skeletal Radiol 1997;26:82–8.
42. Tol JL, Struiss PA, Bossuyt PM, et al. Treatment strategies in osteochondral defects of the talar dome: a systematic review. Foot Ankle Int 2000;21(2):119–26.
43. Nakamae A, Engebretsen L, Bahr R, et al. Natural history of bone bruises after acute knee injury: clinical outcome and histopathological findings. Knee Surg Sports Traumatol Arthrosc 2006;14:1252–8.
44. Shapiro F, Koide S, Glimcher MJ. Cell origin and differentiation in the repair of full-thickness defects of articular cartilage. J Bone Joint Surg Am 1993;75:532–53.
45. Lamb SE, Marsh JL, Hutton JL, et al, Collaborative Ankle Support Trial (CAST Group). Mechanical supports for acute, severe ankle sprain: a pragmatic, multi-centre, randomised controlled trial. Lancet 2009;373(9663):575–81.
46. Kerkhoffs GM, Handoll HH, de Bie R, et al. Surgical versus conservative treatment for acute injuries of the lateral ligament complex of the ankle in adults. Cochrane Database Syst Rev 2007;(2):CD000380.
47. Millington S, Grabner M, Wozelka R, et al. A stereophotographic study of ankle joint contact area. J Orthop Res 2007;25:1465–73.
48. Zengerink M, Szerb I, Hangody L, et al. Current concepts: treatment of osteochondral ankle defects. Foot Ankle Clin 2006;11(2):331–59.
49. van Dijk CN. Management of the sprained ankle. Br J Sports Med 2002;36:83–4.
50. Lyon R, Liu XC, Kubin M, et al. Does extracorporeal shock wave therapy enhance healing of osteochondritis dissecans of the rabbit knee? a pilot study. Clin Orthop Relat Res 2012. [Epub ahead of print].
51. Vulpiani MC, Vetrano M, Trischitta D, et al. Extracorporeal shock wave therapy in early osteonecrosis of the femoral head: prospective clinical study with long-term follow-up. Arch Orthop Trauma Surg 2012;132(4):499–508.
52. Alvarez RG, Cincere B, Channappa C, et al. Extracorporeal shock wave treatment of non- or delayed union of proximal metatarsal fractures. Foot Ankle Int 2011; 32(8):746–54.
53. van der Jagt OP, Piscaer TM, Schaden W, et al. Unfocused extracorporeal shock waves induce anabolic effects in rat bone. J Bone Joint Surg Am 2011;93:38–48.
54. Wang CJ, Wang FS, Yang KD, et al. The effect of shock wave treatment at the tendon-bone interface–an histomorphological and biomechanical study in rabbits. J Orthop Res 2005;23:274–80.
55. Ma HZ, Zeng BF, Li XL, et al. Temporal and spatial expression of BMP-2 in subchondral bone of necrotic femoral heads in rabbits by use of extracorporeal shock waves. Acta Orthop Scand 2008;79:98–105.
56. Wang CJ, Yang KD, Wang FS, et al. Shock wave treatment shows dose-dependent enhancement of bone mass and bone strength after fracture of the femur. Bone 2004;34:225–30.
57. Wang Q, Li ZL, Fu YM, et al. Effect of low-energy shock waves in microfracture holes in the repair of articular cartilage defects in a rabbit model. Chin Med J 2011;124(9):1386–94.
58. Sanchez M, Anitua E, Azofra J, et al. Intra-articular injection of an autologous preparation rich in growth factors for the treatment of knee OA: a retrospective cohort study. Clin Exp Rheumatol 2008;26(5):910–3.

59. Anitua E, Sánchez M, Nurden AT, et al. Platelet-released growth factors enhance the secretion of hyaluronic acid and induce hepatocyte growth factor production by synovial fibroblasts from arthritic patients. Rheumatology 2007;46(12): 1769–72.
60. Mei Dan O, Carmont MR, Laver L, et al. Platelet rich plasma or hyaluronate in the management of osteochondral defects of the talus. Am J Sports Med 2012;40: 534–41.
61. Kon E, Buda R, Filardo G, et al. Platelet-rich plasma: intra-articular knee injections produced favorable results on degenerative cartilage lesions. Knee Surg Sports Traumatol Arthrosc 2010;18:472–9.
62. Engebretsen L, Steffen K, Alsousou J, et al. IOC consensus paper on the use of platelet-rich plasma in sports medicine. Br J Sports Med 2010;44(15):1072–108.
63. Serra CI, Soler C, Carillo JM, et al. Effects of autologous platelet rich plasma on the repair of full thickness articular defects in rabbits. Knee Surg Sports Traumatol Arthrosc 2012. [Epub ahead of print].
64. Weibrich G, Hansen T, Kleis W, et al. Effect of platelet concentration in platelet-rich plasma on peri-implant bone regeneration. Bone 2004;34:665–71.
65. Vidriero EL, Goulding KA, Simon DA, et al. The use of platelet rich plasma in arthroscopy and sports medicine: optimising the healing environment. Arthroscopy 2012;26:269–78.
66. Pache G, Krauss B, Strohm P, et al. Dual-energy CT virtual noncalcium technique: detecting posttraumatic bone marrow lesions–feasibility study. Radiology 2010; 256(2):617–24.
67. Leumann A, Valderrabano V, Plass C, et al. A novel imaging method for osteochondral lesions of the talus–comparison of SPECT-CT with MRI. Am J Sports Med 2011;39:1095–101.

Osteochondral Lesions of the Talus: Defining the Surgical Approach

Navin Verghese, MB.BS (Lond), FRCS (Orth)*, Amy Morgan, MBChB, MRCS,
Anthony Perera, MBChB, FRCS (Orth)

KEYWORDS

• Talus • Osteochondral • Osteotomy • Surgical approaches • Arthroscopy

KEY POINTS

- Preoperative surgical mapping of the site and size of the lesion will enable full exposure to most osteochondral lesions.
- Posterior ankle arthroscopy is required for access to the posterior zones.
- Osteotomies increase the exposure to the talus.
- Medial malleoloar osteotomy is best performed through a step-cut.

INTRODUCTION

Osteochondritis dissecans of the talar dome was first described in 1922 by Kappis. Numerous terms such as osteochondral defect (OCD) and chondral defect are currently used interchangeably to describe this phenomenon of articular cartilage separation that can occur with a varying amount of underlying subchondral bone. The majority of osteochondral lesions of the talus (OLT) are traumatic, usually in an athletic population in the second to fourth decade of life.[1–6] As a consequence, the aim of surgical management is to achieve pain relief and function but in the least invasive way so as to minimize risk and maximize the speed of recovery.

MANAGEMENT OF OSTEOCHONDRAL LESIONS OF THE TALUS

When planning surgery, various factors need to be taken into account, such as the size, depth, and location of the lesion, history of previous surgery, and stage of the disease. All of these factors play an important role in deciding whether to manage conservatively or surgically and, if surgical, the type of procedure and operative approach required.

The types of surgery available to treat OCDs can be conveniently divided into nongrafting and grafting techniques. Nongrafting techniques such as debridement,

Department of Trauma and Orthopaedic Surgery, University Hospital of Wales, Heath Park, Cardiff CF14 4XW, UK
* Corresponding author.
E-mail address: verghesen@cardiff.ac.uk

Foot Ankle Clin N Am 18 (2013) 49–65
http://dx.doi.org/10.1016/j.fcl.2012.12.003
1083-7515/13/$ – see front matter © 2013 Elsevier Inc. All rights reserved.

microfracture, and drilling have been the mainstay of OCD treatment in the knee for decades, and tend to be a good starting point for management of talar OCDs too. The relative technical ease, low cost, and generally good to excellent outcomes make these treatment techniques popular.[7–9] Moreover, access can be minimized. However, in some cases, in particular larger lesions, grafting techniques may be required.[10] Autografts, allografts, and synthetic grafts have all been described, each with their own unique set of advantages and disadvantages. The factor that all the grafting techniques have in common is the need for perpendicular access to the articular surface; nongrafting techniques, on the other hand, allow a far more acute angle of approach. This difference significantly increases the technical difficulty of grafting techniques, especially when considering the tight angles and space available within the ankle joint. Various surgical approaches to the talus have been described in an attempt to negate these difficulties. However, as with all surgical treatments the pathoanatomy needs to be defined preoperatively in order to select the most appropriate surgical procedure and the most appropriate operative approach.

STEP 1: DEFINE THE PATHOLOGY AND SELECT THE SURGICAL PROCEDURE REQUIRED

A variety of classification systems has been used to describe the pathology, most notably that of Berndt and Harty (**Fig. 1**),[11] who classified OLT according to plain radiographic findings. Anderson and colleagues[12] and the later modification by Loomer and colleagues[13] based the classification on computed tomography findings (**Fig. 2**). Canale and Belding[14,15] classified the lesion according to the degree of cartilage damage. The most recent and commonly used classification is that of Hepple and colleagues[16] (**Fig. 3**), who based their grading on magnetic resonance imaging (MRI) findings in a similar fashion to the earlier classification of Berndt and Harty. This description of the pathology determines whether the OLT can be treated with

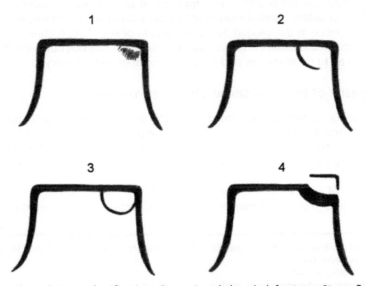

Fig. 1. Berndt and Harty classification. Stage 1: subchondral fracture. Stage 2: partially detached fragment. Stage 3: detached but undisplaced. Stage 4: displaced fragment. (Images reprinted with permission from Medscape Reference (http://emedicine.medscape.com/), 2013, available at: http://emedicine.medscape.com/article/1237723-overview.)

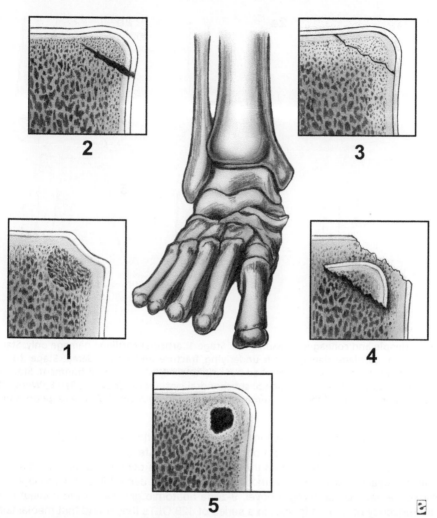

Fig. 2. Computed tomography classification of Anderson and colleagues. Stage 1: subchondral compression (edema). Stage 2: incomplete fracture, undisplaced. Stage 3: complete fracture, undisplaced. Stage 4: displaced fragment. Stage 5 (addition of Loomer and colleagues): radiolucent (fibrous) defect, roof intact. (Images reprinted with permission from Medscape Reference (http://emedicine.medscape.com/), 2013, available at: http://emedicine.medscape.com/article/1237723-overview.)

nongrafting techniques or whether grafting is required, and is therefore the most important initial step in planning the surgical approach.

STEP 2: DEFINE THE ANATOMY AND DETERMINE THE BEST OPERATIVE APPROACH FOR THE SELECTED PROCEDURE

These systems of classification are helpful in determining the best treatment strategy, namely, arthroscopic debridement and microfracture or osteochondral grafting. However, the talus is not accessed as readily as the femoral condyle, and in fact access can be very limited. Therefore, the second step in surgical planning is to

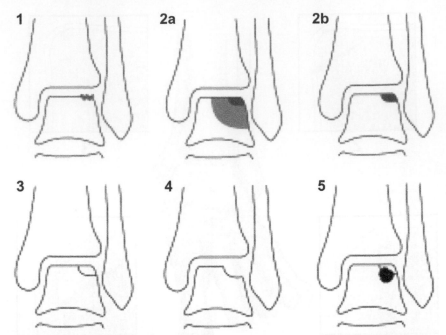

Fig. 3. Hepple and colleagues classification. Stage 1: articular cartilage damage only. Stage 2a: articular cartilage damage with underlying fracture and bony edema. Stage 2b: 2a without bony edema. Stage 3: detached but undisplaced osteochondral fragment. Stage 4: displaced detached fragment. Stage 5: subchondral cyst. (*From* Chew KT, Tay E, Wong YS. Osteochondral lesions of the talus. Ann Acad Med Singapore 2008;37:63–8; with permission.)

determine the anatomy of the OLT in terms of its site on the talus and to plan the operative approach to this area in light of the treatment strategy selected.

Historically it was believed that the majority of OLTs occurred anterolaterally and posteromedially, but this is now thought not to be the case. Elias and colleagues[17] divided the talar dome using a novel, 9-zone anatomic grid system to evaluate the true frequency of OLTs (**Fig. 4**A). In a series of 428 OLTs they found that medial talar dome lesions were both more common and significantly larger than lateral lesions. With regard to specific zones on the talus (**Fig. 4**B), centromedial lesions were the most common, with centrolateral the next most frequent site. Posteromedial and anterolateral lesions were rarely found. These investigators were also able to describe the mean size and depth of these lesions (**Fig. 5**). A prior study by the same group studying MRI changes over time also reported that of 29 OLTs, 19 (66%) were located at the medial talar dome.[18]

ARTHROSCOPIC APPROACHES: NONGRAFTING TECHNIQUES ONLY
Anterior Ankle Arthroscopy

A safe starting point for most OLTs is to perform simple techniques via an arthroscopic approach, hence avoiding the greater morbidity associated with arthrotomy and osteotomy. Most debridement, microfracture, and drilling techniques can be performed via standard anterolateral and anteromedial portals as described by Van Dijk and Scholte.[19] The anteromedial portal is initiated with an 18-gauge spinal needle into the joint. This position is identified by a distinct soft spot usually easily located by

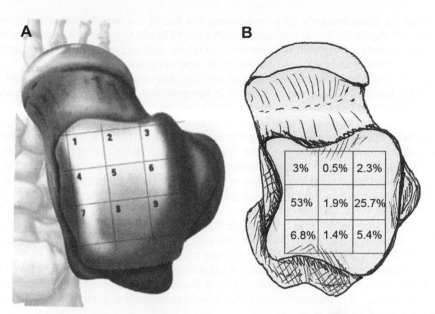

Fig. 4. Talar dome 9-zone grid system of Elias and colleagues.[17] (A) Zone 1 = anteromedial. Zone 9 = posterolateral. (B) Percentage frequency of lesions in each zone.

palpating proximal to distally over the subcutaneous surface of the tibia just medial to the tibialis anterior and feeling for the "step-off" as the joint is reached. The joint capsule is distended by injecting 1% lidocaine with epinephrine to control bleeding. The portal is extended with a no. 11 blade through the skin, and further soft-tissue dissection is performed with a small clamp to avoid injury to the saphenous nerve. A blunt probe is used to penetrate the capsule of the ankle joint. The anterolateral portal is started with a spinal needle that is placed just lateral to the peroneus tertius. This needle should be visualized with the arthroscope via the anteromedial portal to ensure it is suitably placed for instrumentation. Care must be taken to avoid injury to the intermediate branches of the superficial peroneal nerve; the nerve can be

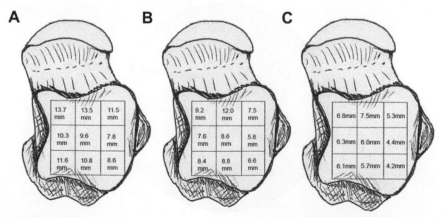

Fig. 5. Dimensions of lesion by zone. (A) Mean anteroposterior size of lesion in each zone. (B) Mean transverse size of lesion in each zone. (C) Mean depth in each zone.

marked out preoperatively by plantarflexing the fourth toe, which makes the nerve prominent. Again the portal is extended with a no. 11 blade and blunt dissection is performed to protect the nerve. The medial and lateral portals can be extended distally and proximally, if necessary, to convert to an open procedure.

Anterior ankle arthroscopy is straightforward and allows excellent access to zones 1, 2, and 3. The access to zones 4, 5, and 6 is more difficult, but with plantarflexion and good distraction debridement of the cartilage is easy, and debridement of the bone is possible with a curved curette (**Fig. 6**). However, it is more difficult to perform microfracture for the more posterior lesions in these zones, owing to the acute angle at which the instruments have to enter the ankle. This problem can be circumvented by performing the microfracture with a K-wire passed retrograde via the lateral process of the talus (**Fig. 7**) or medial talar body, or antegrade via a transmalleolar technique. The transtalar approach is easier and avoids damaging articular cartilage, but it can be difficult to get the K-wire at the correct angle; an instrument needs to be placed over the lesion to prevent the wire penetrating the tibial cartilage. If a transmalleolar approach is to be used, the senior author (A.P.) prefers to drill a 4-mm hole in the outer cortex of the tibia to make it easier for the 2-mm K-wire to pivot around the lesion.

Access to lesions in zones 7, 8, and 9 is extremely limited, and care must be taken to avoid this as it can result in iatrogenic injury at the anterior lip caused by levering of the instrumentation. It is therefore crucial that careful preoperative planning is carried out with the aid of an MRI scan.

Tips

Accessing more posterior lesions requires good plantarflexion, and elevating the leg using a bolster under the thigh can help with this. However, marked plantarflexion and distraction tightens the anterior capsule, and it may be easier to take the distraction off and make the portal a little more superior, allowing a better line of entry as the portal is pulled distally by distraction and plantarflexion.

Posterior Ankle Arthroscopy

In zones 7, 8, and 9 and in more posterior lesions in zones 4, 5, and 6, prone posterior arthroscopy provides a better view and access, especially where nongrafting techniques are to be used. **Fig. 8**[20–22] shows 2 patients with widespread lesions that can only be accessed posteriorly.

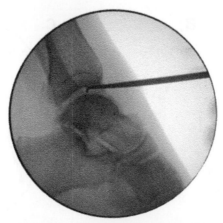

Fig. 6. Accessing zones 4, 5, and 6 via anterior arthroscopy: distraction and plantarflexion. (*Courtesy of* A. Perera, MBChB, FRCS (Orth), Cardiff, UK.)

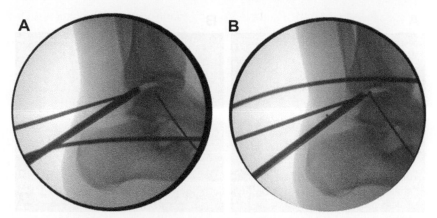

Fig. 7. (*A*) Retrograde K-wire though the lateral process of the talus for microfracture of a posterior talar osteochondral lesion. (*B*) The probe is placed over the lesion to avoid damage to the opposite cortex. (*Courtesy of* A. Perera, MBChB, FRCS (Orth), Cardiff, UK.)

The patient is placed prone with appropriate precautions, and the tourniquet is inflated before the patient is turned. The feet are positioned beyond the end of the table on a gel cushion so that the ankle can be fully dorsiflexed freely by the surgeon. No traction is used, but it is advisable to use a larger, longer 4-mm scope because there is more soft tissue to penetrate than on the anterior side.

The posterolateral portal is based at the midpoint between the posterior border of the fibula and lateral border of the Achilles tendon in the coronal plane. The incision is extended, and blunt dissection is used to protect the sural nerve. The senior author uses the technique described by Van Dijk and Scholte[19] to protect the medial neurovascular bundle; this is swept from lateral to medial using a large clip.

The flexor hallucis longus (FHL) tendon is the crucial marker for the neurovascular bundle, as this lies more medial to the tendon. Dorsiflexion of the ankle provides increased access to the posterior talus.

The posterior process of the talus and zones 7, 8, and 9 are easily visualized with this technique, and posterior parts of zones 4, 5, and 6 can also be accessed (**Fig. 9**). The approach requires greater training and care but is a rewarding procedure to learn. MRI is crucial for preoperative planning. **Fig. 8** shows that the lesion that will be very difficult to treat with anterior arthroscopy, and it is important that this is known before the procedure commences. It is possible to place a posteromedial portal during an anterior arthroscopic procedure, but this is not generally recommended because of its proximity to the posterior tibial artery and nerve.

The exposure to posterior lesions in which grafting techniques may be necessary can be achieved through either posterolateral or posteromedial arthrotomies with or without fibula, or medial malleolar osteotomies. These techniques are described in the next section.

Tips

This technique requires a good course and practice but is rewarding to learn. One must make sure not to stray beyond the FHL tendon to avoid damage to the neurovascular bundle. It is easier to use a 4-mm scope, as it is longer and more rigid. Allow the foot to be far enough off the end of the table, such that full dorsiflexion is possible to allow access to more anterior lesions.

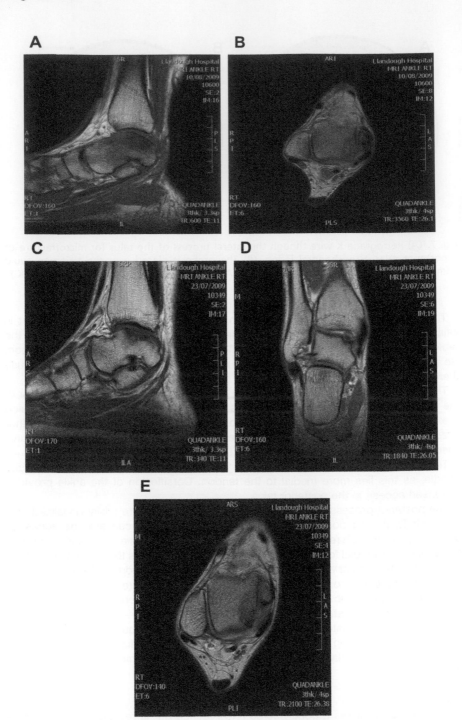

Fig. 8. Posteriotalar lesions in (*A, B*) patient 1 and (*C–E*) patient 2. Both patients show widespread lesions, but the key part lies in zone 9 and can only be accessed from posterior. (*Courtesy of* A. Perera, MBChB, FRCS (Orth), Cardiff, UK.)

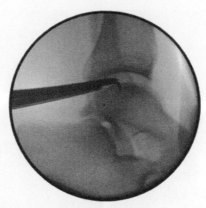

Fig. 9. Posterior arthroscopy to reach the posterior part of zones 4, 5, and 6. It is possible to reach further with dorsiflexion of the ankle. (*Courtesy of* A. Perera, MBChB, FRCS (Orth), Cardiff, UK.)

OPEN APPROACHES TO THE TALUS: NONGRAFTING AND GRAFTING TECHNIQUES

Open techniques can be further subdivided into simple arthrotomy and osteotomy. Cadaveric studies[23] have demonstrated that 75% of the talar dome can be accessed by arthrotomy alone, that medial and lateral malleolar osteotomies allow 100% sagittal exposure, that anterolateral (Chaput tubercle) osteotomy[24] provides additional 22% sagittal lateral exposure, and that with all exposures, 15% of residual area is still inaccessible in the posterior central talar dome. The approach used depends on not only the location of the lesion but also whether nongrafting or grafting techniques are to be used once the lesion is exposed. Nongrafting techniques require far less exposure than grafting techniques whereby a perpendicular path to the lesion is required for implantation. If an osteochondral lesion is of such large size and depth, has failed to respond to arthroscopic techniques, or is in an inaccessible area, open approaches are indicated.

Approaches to the Lateral Talar Dome

Arthrotomy, anterior and posterior
Most lateral talar lesions are central[17] and are accessible via anterolateral arthrotomy because of the posterior location of the fibula in relation to the talus. The incision is centered over the anterolateral ankle using the plane between extensor digitorum longus medially and peroneus tertius laterally. Care must be taken in identifying and protecting the intermediate dorsal cutaneous branches of the superficial peroneal nerve, which are located in this plane. The extensor retinaculum and joint capsule are incised in line with the incision, providing access to the anterolateral talus (**Fig. 10**A). Exposure can further be improved with plantarflexion of the ankle, and in fact gives access to more anterior lesions in zones 6 and lateral 5 very well, which can be further improved by using a distractor (**Fig. 10**B).

Posterolateral OLTs can be accessed via an arthrotomy made between the peroneals and the Achilles tendon, with the patient prone or on his or her side and with the foot free to dorsiflex. The FHL needs to be retracted medially, taking care to avoid injury to the medial neurovascular bundle. Zone 9 is readily seen, and the immediately adjacent zones can be seen with dorsiflexion or medial retraction; however, it is not easy to see much beyond this, and posterior arthroscopy provides greater vision.

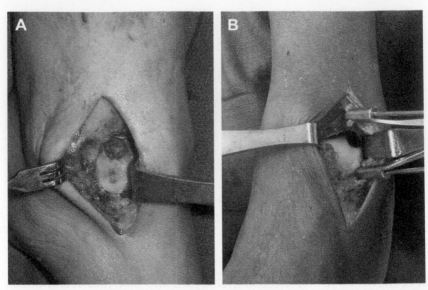

Fig. 10. (*A*) Anterolateral arthrotomy. (*B*) Anterolateral arthrotomy with ankle distraction. (*Courtesy of* Mark S. Myerson, MD, Baltimore, MD.)

Tips A ringed distractor such as a Weinraub or Hinterman distractor allows placement of large smooth K-wires that can increase the distraction across the ankle. Take care when using the posterior approach to protect the neurovascular bundle on the other side of the FHL tendon, particularly with retraction.

Fibular/lateral tibial osteotomy
With larger central or posterolateral lesions requiring grafting, simple arthrotomy may not provide the necessary exposure required for perpendicular access. In these cases fibular osteotomy may be indicated. A longitudinal incision is centered over the distal fibula. Once exposed, the osteotomy is made with a bone-cutting microsaw from proximolateral to distomedial, the distal end being at the level of the joint line. This approach provides an oblique osteotomy with a larger surface area for healing and preservation of the interosseous ligaments. Once the fibula osteotomy has been performed, the lesion can be accessed by simple inversion of the ankle.

More central lesions may require additional lateral distal tibial osteotomy; likewise, some massive anterolateral lesions may require anterolateral distal tibial osteotomy. With all distal tibial osteotomies, one must ensure it is large enough to accept a screw to allow anatomic reduction and compression. The fibula osteotomy is again reduced anatomically and fixed with a lateral plate. Any ligamentous disruption is repaired and, if any disruption of the syndesmosis has occurred, 1 or 2 syndesmosis screws are inserted.

Tips Releasing the syndesmotic and lateral collateral ligaments will increase the exposure, but great care must be taken to ensure an adequate repair.

Approaches to the Medial Talar Dome

Arthrotomy, anterior and posterior
Anteromedial arthrotomies are useful for grafting and nongrafting techniques, especially in the anteromedial zone of the talus; however, this is an uncommon site for

OLTs to be found. A longitudinal incision centered over the joint line using the plane between the tibialis anterior and extensor hallucis longus is developed. Capsulotomy is made in the same orientation as the skin incision. Depending on the exact location of the lesion, the incision and arthrotomy plane can be made medially (ie, between tibialis anterior and the saphenous neurovascular bundle) or laterally (between extensor hallucis longus and extensor digitorum longus).

Posteromedial arthrotomies are more complex and require retraction of the neurovascular bundle, and great care must be taken. However, the view allow grafting of zone 9 and the posterior part of zone 6 (**Fig. 11**).

Tips Ringed distraction, as for anterolateral approaches, can be helpful. Great care must be taken in retraction of the medial neurovascular bundle when using the posteromedial approach. It is difficult to gain perpendicular access to the posteromedial dome, and a medial malleolar osteotomy will often afford a better line of access.

Medial malleolus osteotomy

Unfortunately most medial OLTs lie centrally, and this is a difficult area to access via a simple arthrotomy if grafting techniques are to be used. **Fig. 12** shows a case whereby it was just possible to debride this lesion through anterior arthroscopy and then graft bone through an anteromedial arthrotomy with plantarflexion and curved instruments. However, had bone grafting been required, a formal medial malleolar osteotomy would be required to allow osteochondral grafting perpendicular to the surface.

Medial lesions tend to be more central or posteriorly located, and together with the more anterior position of the medial relative to the lateral malleolus, require medial malleolar osteotomies more frequently than distal fibular osteotomies for lateral lesions. The medial malleolus osteotomy was developed to improve visualization of

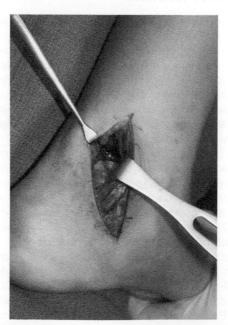

Fig. 11. Retraction of the medial neurovascular bundle and complete osteochondral grafting of the talus. (*Courtesy of* Mark S. Myerson, MD, Baltimore, MD.)

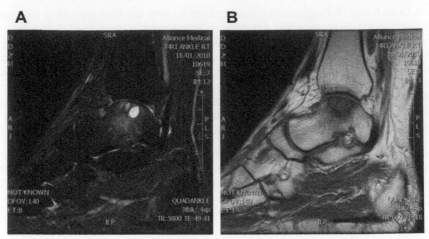

Fig. 12. Medial osteochondral lesion of the talus. (*A*) Fluid sensitive MRI sequence. (*B*) T1 MRI sequence. (*Courtesy of* A. Perera, MBChB, FRCS (Orth), Cardiff, UK.)

the talus. For talar body fractures and osteochondral lesions of the talar dome, straight and step-cut osteotomy techniques have been described.[25–28]

Tips The tibialis posterior tendon is closely opposed to the posteromedial tibia, and care must be taken to avoid damage to this key structure. The retinaculum can be released, and a Trethowan retractor can be applied to the bone underneath the tendon. Step-cut osteotomies are more stable and heal better than straight-cut osteotomies.

STRAIGHT-CUT OSTEOTOMY TECHNIQUE

Straight cuts can either be transverse or oblique, entering the joint at the level of the axilla of the medial malleolus.[26–28] Oblique osteotomies are more useful for OLTs, and it is useful to line up the osteotomy using an image-guided 2-mm K-wire that can act as a jig for the saw to ensure that sufficient exposure is achieved.

The skin incision is centered over the medial malleolus.[25] Periosteum is reflected anteriorly and posteriorly approximately 1.5 cm proximal to the joint line. Tibialis posterior tendon is identified and protected at all times. A 2-mm K-wire is passed into the joint, skirting the axilla to provide a reference point (**Fig. 13**A), which can be used as a guide for the saw blade.

An incomplete saw cut is made and this is finished using an osteotome. Care must be taken to protect the tibialis posterior tendon, as this can be injured. The osteotomy will be secured back in place with a lag screw at the end of the procedure. The medial malleolus should therefore be predrilled at this stage before osteotomy to ensure anatomic reduction and optimal fixation of the osteotomy fragment afterward (**Fig. 13**B), done with 2 parallel extra-articular drill holes in a similar direction and location to standard medial malleolar fracture fixation lag screws.

After the intra-articular procedure is completed, the medial malleolus is placed back into anatomic position using the anteromedial joint line as a guide. It is secured with 2 partially threaded 4.0-mm cancellous lag screws[25] (**Fig. 13**C). Postoperatively the patient is started with early ankle motion to improve cartilage healing when the incision is healed adequately. Protected weight-bearing using either a cast or a fracture boot is allowed after 2 weeks, and unprotected weight-bearing is begun at 6 weeks if radiographic and clinical examinations indicate adequate healing.[25]

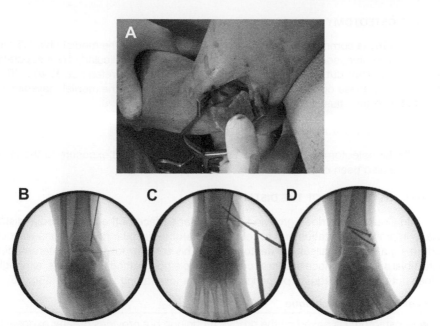

Fig. 13. Medial malleolus straight-cut osteotomy technique. (*A*) Intraoperative photograph demonstrating excellent perpendicular access to the talar dome achieved after osteotomy has been completed. (*B*) K-wire placed in axilla as reference. (*C*) Predrilling prior to osteotomy. (*D*) Osteotomy fragment lagged with × 2 4.0 mm partially threaded cancellous screws after grafting has been completed. (*Courtesy of* Mark S. Myerson, MD, Baltimore, MD; A. Perera, MBChB, FRCS (Orth), Cardiff, UK.)

Straight osteotomies, however, lack interdigitation, and even with predrilling of the malleolus this can result in rotation and subsequent malunion and incongruence of the articular surface of the malleolus (**Fig. 14**A). Because of this problem, step-cut osteotomies are recommended, providing more stability and resistance to rotation (**Fig. 14**B, C).

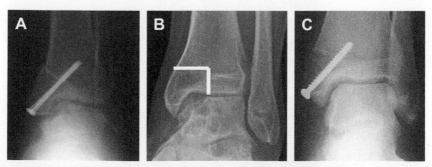

Fig. 14. (*A*) Malunited medial malleolus osteotomy. (*B*) Planned approach to a centromedial OLT. (*C*) Healed step-cut osteotomy. ([*A*] *From* Navid DO, Myerson MS. Approach alternatives for treatment of osteochondral lesions of the talus. Foot Ankle Clin 2002;7(3):635–49. [*B*] *Courtesy of* A. Perera, MBChB, FRCS (Orth), Cardiff, UK. [*C*] *From* Amendola A, Panarella L. Osteochondral lesions: medial versus lateral, persistent pain, cartilage restoration options and indications. Foot Ankle Clin 2009;14:215–27.)

STEP-CUT OSTEOTOMY TECHNIQUE

The osteotomy is commenced with a transverse saw cut into the medial tibia 1.5 cm above the joint line (see **Fig. 14**B, C). This cut is met perpendicularly by a separate osteotome sagittal cut directed vertically upwards from the reference K-wire. The depths of both these cuts should be equal. When separated, the medial malleolus is retracted, and the talus is exposed.

DISTAL TIBIAL INTRA-ARTICULAR OSTEOTOMIES

Nonmalleolar osteotomies of the distal tibia to allow increased exposure to the talar dome have also been described.[29–36]

CHANNEL OSTEOTOMY OF THE DISTAL TIBIA

Flick and Gould[29] described grooving the articular surface of the anteromedial distal tibia to improve visualization and access to posteromedial talar dome lesions without performing a medial malleolus osteotomy.[29,35] This small groove in the anteromedial distal tibial articular surface allows access for simple nongrafting techniques, although it does not provide adequate perpendicular paths for grafting procedures (**Fig. 15**).

Channel Osteotomy Technique

Channel osteotomy is based on the groove technique but provides greater exposure, hence allowing for grafting techniques to be performed.[35] In the channel technique, the distal tibia is osteotomized in such a manner as to remove a block of distal tibia in line with the talar lesion. When this bone is removed temporarily, the area of missing bone creates a channel leading directly to the talar dome. This technique is particularly useful for posterolateral talar dome lesions.

A standard anterolateral arthrotomy is performed as described previously. The talar dome is plantarflexed fully to determine if the osteochondral lesion can be exposed. If it cannot, such as in large central or posterolateral lesions, a channel osteotomy will be required. Based on the location of the lesion on preoperative imaging and direct

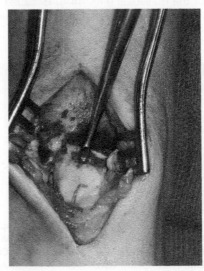

Fig. 15. Grooving of the tibia to improve access. (*Courtesy of* Mark S. Myerson, MD, Baltimore, MD.)

intraoperative visualization, a section of periosteum is reflected from the distal antero-lateral tibia in line with the lesion.

A rectangular area, 15 mm width and 25 mm in length, is marked on the anterior tibia at the correct location, with the longer lines oriented in the sagittal plane and the shorter line oriented transversely. The tibial plafond acts as the inferior border of the rectangle. A sagittal saw is used to initiate the cuts through the distal tibia. The superior cut should be angled 30° to 45° downward so that the cut extends posterior and distal toward the articular surface. To prevent significant articular cartilage loss, the cuts are completed with an osteotome through the subchondral bone and joint surface. The resultant triangular block of bone and cartilage is removed and kept wrapped in a moist sponge to prevent desiccation. The resulting "channel" defect in the distal tibia allows visualization of the talar dome lesion. Grafting techniques can now be performed with perpendicular access to the lesion. After the lesion has been addressed the osteotom-ized bone is reduced anatomically, and fixed with K-wires or lagged with screws. Fluo-roscopy is used to verify correct replacement of the osteotomy.

DISTAL TIBIAL PLAFONDPLASTY

Anterior distal tibial plafondplasty as described by Peters and colleagues[36] is based on the same principles as the channel osteotomy. A triangular wedge of distal tibia either anterolaterally or medially is fashioned in much the same way as described for the channel osteotomy. Peters and colleagues described smaller wedges of 10 by 10 mm with cut angles of 30° to 40° toward the articular surface. Objectively, however, they compared plafondplasty with standard anterolateral and anteromedial arthrotomies on cadavers, and demonstrated significantly increased talar dome expo-sure with plafondplasty. It was possible to increase the sagittal access by more than 50% in comparison with arthrotomy alone. Only the central posterior 10% of the dome was not accessible by this method, so the investigators suggested that distal tibial plafondplasty may be used in the majority of cases hence avoiding medial or lateral malleolar osteotomies. However, with appropriate planning this area can also be visualized (**Fig. 16**).

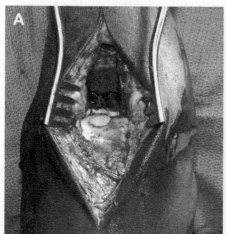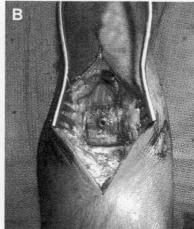

Fig. 16. Access to the central zones via an anterior plafondplasty. (A) after removal of wedge of anterior tibial plafond. graft in situ. (B) tibial plafond wedge restored and lagged with dual compression screw. (*Courtesy of* Mark S. Myerson, MD, Baltimore, MD.)

REFERENCES

1. Konig F. Veber freie Korper in der Gelenken. Dtsch Z Chir 1888;27:90–109.
2. Giannini S, Buda R, Grigolo B, et al. Autologous chondrocyte transplantation in osteochondral lesions of the ankle joint. Foot Ankle Int 2004;22(6):168–75.
3. Navid DO, Myerson MS. Approach alternatives for treatment of osteochondral lesions of the talus. Foot Ankle Clin 2002;7(3):635–49.
4. Bosien WR, Staples OS, Russell SW. Residual disability following ankle sprains. J Bone Joint Surg Am 1955;37-A:1237–43.
5. Dipaola JD, Nelson DW, Colville MR. Characterizing osteochondral lesions by magnetic resonance imaging. Arthroscopy 1991;7:101–4.
6. Farmer JM, Martin DF, Boles CA, et al. Chondral and osteochondral injuries. Diagnosis and management. Clin Sports Med 2001;20:299–320.
7. Stetson WB, Ferkel RD. Ankle arthroscopy: II. Indications and results. J Am Acad Orthop Surg 1996;4:24–34.
8. Tol JL, Struijs PA, Bossuyt PM, et al. Treatment strategies in osteochondral defects of the talar dome: a systematic review. Foot Ankle Int 2000;21:119–26.
9. Verhagen RA, Struijs PA, Bossuyt PM, et al. Systematic review of treatment strategies for osteochondral defects of the talar dome. Foot Ankle Clin 2003;8:233–42, viii–ix.
10. Lynn AK, Brooks RA, Bonfield W, et al. Repair of defects in articular joints. Prospects for material-based solutions in tissue engineering. J Bone Joint Surg Br 2004;86:1093–9. Available at: http://dx.doi.org/10.1302/0301-620X.86B8.15609. Accessed April 1, 2012.
11. Berndt AL, Harty M. Transchondral fractures (osteochondritis dissecans) of the talus. J Bone Joint Surg Am 1959;41-A:988–1020.
12. Anderson IF, Crichton KJ, Grattan-Smith T, et al. Osteochondral fractures of the dome of the talus. J Bone Joint Surg Am 1989;71:1143–52.
13. Loomer R, Fisher C, Lloyd-Smith R, et al. Osteochondral lesions of the talus. Am J Sports Med 1993;21:13–9.
14. Canale ST, Belding RH. Osteochondral lesions of the talus. J Bone Joint Surg Am 1980;62:97–102.
15. Pritsch M, Horoshovski H, Farine I. Arthroscopic treatment of osteochondral lesions of the talus. J Bone Joint Surg Am 1986;68:862–5.
16. Hepple S, Winson IG, Glew D. Osteochondral lesions of the talus: a revised classification. Foot Ankle Int 1999;20:789–93.
17. Elias I, Zoga AC, Morrison WB, et al. Osteochondral lesions of the talus: localization and morphologic data from 424 patients using a novel anatomical grid scheme. Foot Ankle Int 2007;28(2):154–61.
18. Elias I, Jung JW, Raikin SM, et al. Osteochondral lesions of the talus: change in MRI findings over time in talar lesions without operative intervention and implications for staging systems. Foot Ankle Int 2006;27(3):157–66.
19. Van Dijk CN, Scholte D. Arthroscopy of the ankle joint. Arthroscopy 1997;13(1):90–6.
20. Phisitkul P, Junko J, Femino JE, et al. Techniques of prone ankle and subtalar arthroscopy. Tech Foot Ankle Surg 2007;6:30–7.
21. Phisitkul P, Tochigi Y, Saltzman CL, et al. Arthroscopic visualization of the posterior subtalar joint in the prone position: a cadaver study. Arthroscopy 2006;22:511–5.
22. Sitler DF, Amendola A, Bailey CS, et al. Posterior ankle arthroscopy: an anatomic study. J Bone Joint Surg Am 2002;84-A:763–9.

23. Muir D, Saltzman CL, Tochigi Y, et al. Talar dome access for osteochondral lesions. Am J Sports Med 2006;34:1457–63.
24. Tochigi Y, Amendola A, Muir D, et al. Surgical approach for centrolateral talar osteochondral lesions with an anterolateral osteotomy. Foot Ankle Int 2002;23:1038–9.
25. Alexander I, Watson T. Step-cut osteotomy of the medial malleolus for exposure of the medial ankle joint space. Foot Ankle Int 1991;11:242.
26. Crenshaw AH. Surgical techniques. In: Edmonson AS, Crenshaw AH, editors. Campbell's operative orthopaedics. 6th edition. St Louis (MO): CV Mosby; 1980.
27. Mayo KA. Fractures of the talus: principles of management and techniques of treatment. Tech Orthop 1987;2:42.
28. Ove PN, Bosse MJ, Reinert CM, et al. Excision of posterolateral talar dome lesions through a medial transmalleolar approach. Foot Ankle 1989;9:171.
29. Flick AB, Gould N. Osteochondritis dissecans of the talus (transchondral fractures of the talus): review of the literature and new surgical approach for medial dome lesions. Foot Ankle 1985;5:165–85.
30. Ly PN, Fallat LM. Trans-chondral fractures of the talus: a review of 64 surgical cases. J Foot Ankle Surg 1993;32:352–74.
31. McCullough CJ, Venugopal V. Osteochondritis dissecans of the talus: the natural history. Clin Orthop 1979;144:264–8.
32. Pettine KA, Morrey BF. Osteochondral fractures of the talus: a long-term followup. J Bone Joint Surg Br 1987;69:89–92.
33. Shea MP, Manoli A. Osteochondral lesions of the talar dome. Foot Ankle 1993;14:48–55.
34. Thordason DB. Talar body fractures. Orthop Clin N Am 2001;32:65–77.
35. Mangone PG. Distal tibial osteotomies for the treatment of foot and ankle disorders. Foot Ankle Clin 2001;6:3.
36. Peters PG, Parks BG, Schon LC. Anterior distal tibia plafondplasty for exposure of the talar dome. Foot Ankle Int 2012;33:3.

Osteochondral Lesion of the Talus
Prognostic Factors Affecting the Clinical Outcome After Arthroscopic Marrow Stimulation Technique

Woo Jin Choi, MD, Joon Jo, MD, Jin Woo Lee, MD, PhD*

KEYWORDS

- Osteochondral lesion of talus (OLT) • Microfracture • Age • Subchondral cyst • Size
- Location • Containment

KEY POINTS

- Many factors, including age, defect size, location, and the presence of a cyst, should be considered when treating patients with osteochondral lesions of the talus (OLTs).
- Increasing age is not an independent risk factor for poor clinical outcome after the arthroscopic treatment of OLTs.
- In patients with a large area of more than 150 mm^2, the clinical failure rate was significantly higher.
- The existence of a cyst in osteochondral defects might not affect the postoperative prognosis.
- Patients with an uncontained lesion experienced inferior clinical outcomes as compared with patients with a contained lesion after arthroscopic treatment.
- Osteochondral transplantation is a viable alternative secondary procedure for treating unstable OLTs that are refractive to arthroscopic treatment.

Osteochondral lesions of the talus (OLTs) involving talar articular cartilage and subchondral bone are common injuries often found in patients with chronic disabling pain after ankle sprains.[1,2] There were numerous theories concerning the underlying cause of OLTs, including traumatic, vascular, endocrine or metabolic, degenerative joint disease, and genetic causes.[1,3–13] A traumatic insult is more widely accepted as the cause of OLTs, usually in the form of ankle sprains.[1,8–14] A severe ankle sprain can cause a small fracture and subsequent impaired vascularity, leading to the formation of an osteochondral defect. In addition, microtrauma caused by repetitive articular cartilage surface loading or excessive stress can lead to cellular degeneration or death by the disruption of collagen fibril ultrastructure and thickening of the subchondral bone.[15]

Department of Orthopaedic Surgery, Yonsei University College of Medicine, Seoul 120-752, South Korea
* Corresponding author.
E-mail address: ljwos@yuhs.ac

Foot Ankle Clin N Am 18 (2013) 67–78
http://dx.doi.org/10.1016/j.fcl.2012.12.004
1083-7515/13/$ – see front matter © 2013 Elsevier Inc. All rights reserved.

foot.theclinics.com

OLTs that are asymptomatic or discovered as nondisplaced can be treated with conservative treatments in both children and adults. Surgical treatment of OLTs is reserved for symptomatic focal lesions that fail to respond to conservative treatments. Asymptomatic lesions are usually followed with serial radiographs. Chronic lesions or lesions that remain symptomatic despite a trial of conservative measures should be considered for surgical treatment. Furthermore, lesions that are identified incidentally or that are not confirmed to be the source of the symptoms should be managed with nonsurgical measures. In children, cartilage damage with lower-grade OLT cases can be cured with conservative treatment. However, these cases are not common in adult patients.[16,17] Patients who are asymptomatic or nondisplaced with lesions only in the cartilage can be treated nonoperatively with rest, ice, temporarily reduced weight bearing, and, in the case of ankle malalignment, an orthosis. Other possible options include non–weight-bearing treatment with cast immobilization, protected weight bearing in a walking boot, bracing, physical therapy, and nonsteroidal antiinflammatory drugs. If healing is in process, conservative treatment will continue until symptom free; but if it is not, patients may have to find other treatment options. The reason OLTs produce symptoms is poorly understood. It has been theorized that a focal loss of structural support of the talar dome or a cyclical change in intraosseous pressure with gait activates pain receptors in the highly innervated subchondral bone.[18] A thorough examination of the ankle and hindfoot should be performed to identify other potential causes of ankle pain and identify other associated pathologic conditions, including soft tissue impingement, synovitis, and syndesmosis widening.[19,20]

OPERATIVE TREATMENT OPTIONS

The principal aim of surgical treatment is revascularization of the bony defect.[21–25] Because articular hyaline cartilage is avascular and has poor regenerative capabilities, injuries that do not penetrate the subchondral plate have no stimulus for an inflammatory reaction. The category of surgical treatment can be compressed into 3 areas.[12,26–28]

1. Debridement and bone marrow stimulation, with or without loose body removal (microfracture, abrasion chondroplasty, curettage, or antegrade drilling)
2. Securing a lesion to the talar dome (retrograde drilling, bone grafting, or internal fixation)
3. Stimulating the development of hyaline cartilage (osteochondral autografts [mosaicplasty], allografts, or autologous chondrocyte implantation [ACI])

Most cartilage lesions can be treated and approximated by arthroscopy. Arthroscopic treatment is often performed on an outpatient basis and carries the theoretical benefits of limited surgical morbidity, decreased stiffness, less muscle atrophy, shorter rehabilitation times, and improved functional outcomes. In Parisien's[12] comprehensive report on ankle arthroscopy techniques, he described portal approaches for synovectomy, debridement, loose body removal, curettage, abrasion, and drilling in the treatment of OLTs. The 88% excellent and satisfactory results have been confirmed by the experience of Van Buecken and colleagues[8] and others[29–31] who have promoted wide and modified use of these techniques.

DEBRIDEMENT AND MICROFRACTURE

Microfracture was designed initially for patients with a posttraumatic or degenerative OTL that had progressed to a full-thickness chondral defect. This technique is a kind of bone marrow–stimulation technique including an abrasion chondroplasty, curettage, and antegrade drilling. Before stimulating the marrow, the lesion is inspected arthroscopically. Arthroscopic findings regarding the viability of the fragment to determine whether or not a lesion can be left untreated, debrided, or microfractured have been described.[32] If the articular cartilage shows minimal fraying or chondromalacia with good stability of the fragment, simple debridement or radiofrequency ablation can be performed without microfracture. When unstable, advanced fraying or softening of the lesion is present, debridement with the marrow stimulation technique is indicated. Like other procedures, a microfracture using an awl to stimulate the release of cells and cytokines from the marrow to heal an OLT has been described in the literature. When an unstable cartilage flap and fragment that overlie subchondral bone is diagnosed and primary fixation is thought to be impossible, removal of the loose body and debridement of the bony bed are indicated. The base of the bed should be debrided back to bleeding bone, and the edges should be located in healthy cartilage. This technique is designed to penetrate the subchondral bone to fill the debrided talar lesion with blood-containing precursor cells and cytokines that will mediate a healing response to form fibrin clot and fibrocartilaginous repair tissue. These tissues have been studied extensively and are mainly comprised of type I collagen, whereas hyaline cartilage consists primarily of type II collagen.[33,34] Although fibrocartilage poses an advantage over exposed subchondral bone as a surface for weight bearing, it has been shown to have inferior stiffness, resilience, and wear properties as compared with normal hyaline cartilage.[35] These techniques have been used to treat lesions of all grades and sizes. The authors have found that arthroscopic debridement accompanied by microfracture of the subchondral bone is a reliable and repeatable procedure to stimulate the biologic repair of the cartilage lesion of the talus in patients in whom nonoperative treatment has failed or in whom acute lesions were encountered during an arthroscopy. They have been used as the initial treatment and as the secondary option following failure of a previous procedure.

Although there have been successful studies reported of platelet-rich plasma (PRP) or bone morphogenic protein (BMP) being transplanted into animal osteochondral defects, reported clinical outcomes are limited. The reason for the overall failure to consistently form hyalinelike repair cartilage using growth factor–based techniques requires further investigation. Factors involved can be broadly described as issues to do with appropriate differentiation of the mesenchymal stem cells (MSCs), loss of transplanted PRP or BMP, degradation of implanted matrices, and failure to integrate with native tissue. With the growth factor–based repair techniques, it is still not clear where the cells that constitute the repair tissue have originated from, whether they are made from PRP or migrated from subchondral bone marrow or adjacent tissue during the repair process. Before growth factor–based cartilage repair can be used clinically, these issues need to be addressed.

PROGNOSTIC FACTORS AFFECTING CLINICAL OUTCOME

Although an OLT is a common cause of chronic ankle pain and disability, the analyses of the clinical features of predictive values, such as age, sex, duration of symptoms, location, and size of the cartilage defect, have been inconsistent and unsatisfactory.[4,36,37] Several recent studies have indicated that older patients seem to do well with an arthroscopic treatment of OLTs,[20,38–40] whereas others have reported a less favorable outcome in older patients.[41–43] Across several series, predictors of worse possible outcomes of arthroscopic treatment include the presence and severity of associated lesions as well as the size of the cartilage defect.[23,41,42,44–46] However, these variables have traditionally been assessed with plain radiographs or during arthroscopic surgery. Many surgeons have recommended various treatment modalities for subchondral cysts of the talus, and the treatment results for subchondral cystic lesions were controversial in previous reports.[40,47–49] The relative prognostic significance of the containment and location of OLTs remains controversial. Most previous studies have addressed the prognostic significance of the containment and location separately, and the conclusions have often been conflicting.[50–52]

It has been the authors' experience that the problem of a persistent or recurrent symptom after a previous arthroscopic treatment is often complicated by a myriad of responsible prognostic factors that may result in unpredictable outcomes. The authors' hypotheses are the following: (1) Increasing age is not an independent risk factor for poor clinical outcome after arthroscopic treatment of OLTs; therefore, age alone should not be a contraindication for arthroscopic treatment. (2) Preoperative measurement of an initial defect size using magnetic resonance imaging (MRI) provides valuable prognostic information about the clinical outcome of OLT. There is a cutoff point regarding the risk of clinical failure at a defect area of approximately 150 mm^2 as calculated from MRI. (3) An OLT with the subchondral cyst (less than 1.5 cm^2) can be treated by arthroscopic procedures without bone grafting, and the existence of a cyst in an osteochondral defect might not affect a postoperative prognosis. (4) The identification of the containment of an OLT by preoperative MRI provides useful prognostic information. Patients with a shoulder-type OLT experience a worse clinical outcome as compared with patients with a non–shoulder-type OLT regardless of location, even after adjustment for OLT size.

This review summarizes the factors influencing the clinical outcomes of OLT when the arthroscopic bone marrow–stimulation technique is performed based on all current research and the authors' experiences.

Age

Many previous studies have reported about the correlation between age and clinical outcomes after an arthroscopic treatment of OLTs. Cuttica and colleagues[53] retrospectively evaluated a total of 130 patients. They reported that age seems to play a role in the clinical outcome and that there was a small increase in the risk of a poor outcome as age progressed up to 33 years. Deol and colleagues[54] reported that prognosis is good or excellent in patients younger than 20 years. Also, some previous studies demonstrated a significant difference in the clinical outcome depending on age after arthroscopic treatment with microfracture for osteochondral defect on the knee.[43,55–57] On the other hand, other studies exhibited different results. They reported no significant relationship between different age groups, but they lacked the evidence to demonstrate a statistical difference because of a small number of patients.[31,40–42]

The authors evaluated the effect of age on the long-term outcome of patients after arthroscopic treatment of OLTs.[19] In contrast to previous studies, the authors' study is unique in that it analyzed 6 different age groups: younger than 20 years, 20 to 29 years, 30 to 39 years, 40 to 49 years, 50 to 59 years, and 60 years and older. The authors' study showed that older age is not an independent predictor for clinical failure after arthroscopic treatment of OLTs. The authors have found that older patients were less likely to have a history of trauma and had a longer duration of symptoms, smaller osteochondral defects, and had more associated intra-articular lesions. Based on these results, the authors assumed that patients are less likely to get injured from outdoor activities as they get older. Likewise, the size of the osteochondral defect decreased as patient age increased. The authors only hypothesized that younger patients were more exposed to sports activities than older patients, and it is this increased exposure that is what causes younger patients to be more likely to have larger osteochondral defects. In previous in vitro studies that reported an age-related decline in the number of MSCs in the bone marrow,[58–61] most of the decline occurred before 30 years of age, with little or no change thereafter. This finding is in accordance with the authors' hypothesis that MSCs from aged patients maintain normal functional capacity and that there is either no age-related effects on MSCs or even an age-related increase in MSCs.[61–64] For this reason, age alone should not be a contraindication for arthroscopic treatment; it is important for surgeons to recognize that older and younger patients had similar clinical outcomes. It will be important to develop algorithms that can carefully select older patients with OLTs who are good candidates for arthroscopic treatment and young patients with large OLTs for osteochondral transplantation to optimize their outcomes.

Defect Size

Across several series, predictors of the worse possible outcomes of arthroscopic treatment include the presence and severity of associated lesions as well as the size of the cartilage defect.[23,41,42,44–46] Many previous investigators mentioned the correlation between defect size and clinical outcome. Christensen and colleagues[65] presented the contact characteristics of ankle joints in 18 fresh cadaver specimens using pressure-sensitive film. The results suggested that the size of the lesion may alter contact stresses in the ankle and that statistically significant changes in contact characteristics occur with lesions larger than 7.5 × 15.0 mm. They concluded that this finding suggests that the size of a lesion is a prognostic factor in patients with a cartilage defect. Giannini and colleagues[66] reported that a lesion less than 150 mm^2 should be treated by an arthroscopic procedure for the first time. However, a patient with a lesion larger than 150 mm^2 or with failed previous surgery should be treated with an osteochondral autogenous graft or ACI. Gobbi and colleagues[23] demonstrated an inverse relationship between the size of a chondral lesion and the clinical outcome. Chuckpaiwong and colleagues[41] and Cuttica and colleagues[53] reported that OLTs larger than 15 mm show a strong correlation with a poor clinical outcome regardless of age, body mass index, previous injury, and the location of lesion.

In the authors' previous study,[34] 120 ankles had an arthroscopic bone marrow–stimulation procedure performed for OLT and the defect size was evaluated as a prognostic factor. Only 3 out of 58 ankles (5.2%) with a defect area less than 100 mm^2 showed clinical failure, likewise for 7 out of 37 ankles (18.9%) with an area between 100 mm^2 and 150 mm^2, whereas the clinical failure rate was significantly higher in patients with an area greater than 150 mm^2 (80%, 20 out of 25) (**Fig. 1**). The results suggested that the marrow-stimulation technique reduces weight stress on the area of cartilage repair and redistributes weight bearing to other less fragile tissues in smaller-sized defects. However, for larger defects, the redistribution of weight bearing is a disadvantage because increased stress could occur and cause damage in some regions of healthy cartilage, which may explain why patients with large lesions have yielded poor outcomes and why marrow-stimulation techniques did not adequately redistribute weight in those cases. The defect size is one of the strongest prognostic factors after an arthroscopic marrow-stimulation technique for OLTs. Treatment algorithms enlist arthroscopic microfracture as a first-line option for therapy of borderline OLTs with osteochondral grafting as an alternative. It remains imperative that one focuses on patient-specific and defect-specific variables, which should guide tailored treatment options for every individual.

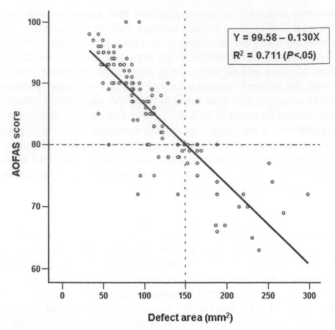

Fig. 1. Correlation between defect size and clinical outcome. (*From* Choi WJ, Park KK, Kim BS, et al. Osteochondral lesion of the talus: is there a critical defect size for poor outcome? Am J Sports Med 2009;37(10):1974–80; with permission.)

Subchondral Cyst

With the development of new diagnostic tools, the classification criteria were revised using a computed tomography or MRI. Anderson and colleagues[9] and Hepple and colleagues[47] proposed a new staging system that included a subchondral cystic lesion of the talus as stage IIA and V (**Fig. 2**). The theories of the pathogenesis of these cystic lesions have been postulated. One involves an intrusion of synovial fluid or herniation of the synovial membrane into the bone through articular defects. According to this theory, a chondral fracture extending through the underlying subchondral bony plate results in a buildup of pressure from the forceful entry of synovial fluid and subsequent cyst formations. Another theory involves mucoid degeneration of

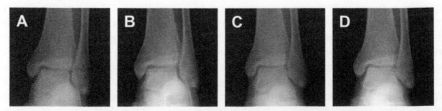

Fig. 2. An anteroposterior radiograph before an operation (*A*) and 1 month (*B*), 6 months (*C*), and 2 years (*D*) after an operation. The medial radiolucent area is a cystic lesion of the talus. A decreased cyst size and increment of density is seen in serial follow-up radiograph. (*From* Han SH, Lee JW, Lee DY, et al. Radiographic changes and clinical results of osteochondral defects of the talus with and without subchondral cysts. Foot Ankle Int 2006;27(12):1109–14; with permission.)

intramedullary connective tissue, probably preceded by focal ischemia or aseptic necrosis.[67–69]

The authors compared the radiographic changes and clinical results in small subchondral talar cystic lesions (less than 150 mm^2) with other noncystic defects after an arthroscopic bone marrow–stimulation procedure without bone grafting.[46] In an analysis between radiological and clinical results, the authors found that the results showed no difference in the clinical outcome between the cystic and noncystic lesion. Furthermore, the authors found good results after arthroscopic treatment of OLT with a small subchondral cystic lesion. Thus, the authors concluded that small cystic lesions can be treated by an arthroscopic marrow-stimulation procedure without bone graft and that the presence of cysts in the OLT will not affect postoperative clinical outcomes.

Containment and Location

The relative prognostic significance of the containment and location of OLT has been of considerable dispute. The usefulness and validity of distinguishing OLTs by containment of the cartilage defect on the talar dome continues to be debated, although in osteochondritis dissecans of the knee joint, clear differences in the clinical outcomes of lesions with contained and uncontained cartilage defects are acknowledged.[70,71] Schimmer and colleagues[72] have suggested that patients with a medial OLT have a better outcome than patients with a lateral OLT. In a study of 44 athletic patients with OLT, Saxena and Eakin[73] noted that patients with an anterolateral OLT had a quicker return-to-activity time and high American Orthopaedic Foot and Ankle Society scores as compared with those with a medial OLT after a microfracture and autogenous bone graft. Chuckpaiwong and colleagues[41] recently mentioned that medial OLTs had a statistically significant correlation with a successful outcome, although they did not distinguish patients by containment (shoulder-type vs non–shoulder-type). However, multivariate analysis in this study of 105 cases indicated that the difference in clinical outcome between patients with medial and lateral OLTs was caused by a larger size of the lateral OLTs and not to the location having an independent prognostic effect. But others have observed no evidence to support the difference in outcome based on the location of the lesions.[20,31] Cuttica and colleagues[53] concluded that the containment and defect size should be considered prognostic factors because an uncontained and larger lesion often revealed inferior functional outcomes. The investigators of that study explained that uncontained lesions lack a stable border for the formation of fibrocartilage after bone marrow stimulation.

The authors evaluated 399 ankles that underwent arthroscopic marrow stimulation for OLTs to determine prognostic factors for clinical outcome. A contained lesion was defined as a cartilage defect that involved the surrounding articular cartilage, whereas an uncontained lesion did not have a peripheral cartilage border (Fig. 3). Contained lesions entailed the non–shoulder-type, whereas uncontained lesions comprised the shoulder-type. Analyses were performed by grouping the patients according to the type of containment (shoulder-type, n = 181; non–shoulder-type, n = 218), location (medial, n = 274; lateral, n = 125), and both type of containment and location (medial shoulder, n = 129; medial non–shoulder-type, n = 145; lateral shoulder-type, n = 52; lateral non–shoulder-type, n = 73). Patients with a shoulder-type OLT had a substantially worse clinical outcome compared with those with a non–shoulder-type OLT, even after adjustment for OLT size. However, there was no significant difference in clinical outcome between patients with medial OLTs and those with lateral OLTs; the clinical failure rates of the two groups were similar. The authors' results indicate that the containment type of OLTs (shoulder-type vs non–shoulder-type) is of greater

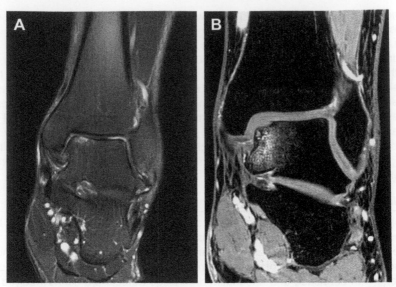

Fig. 3. Coronal images of magnetic resonance imaging show that an osteochondral lesion of the medial dome of the talus. (*A*) Contained, non–shoulder-type. (*B*) Uncontained, shoulder-type.

prognostic significance as compared with the OLT location (medial vs lateral), independent of OLT size.

The authors think that a small lesion with an intact cartilage border provides space during the loading of the ankle joint and the undifferentiated MSCs migrate into the clot filling the chondral defect, or their subsequent proliferation and differentiation into at least fibrocartilage tissue, whereas when a lesion is too large or margin is not intact, joint loading leads to the compression of the material filling the defect and the disruption of cartilage repair. In microfracture procedures, fibrocartilage is inherently unstable and will shear off in an uncontained lesion. Furthermore, in open reconstructive procedures, cartilage cells cannot adequately restore the contour of the talar shoulder. Therefore, a more detailed investigation and an advanced surgical procedure with tissue-engineered scaffolds may be warranted in patients with an uncontained OLT shoulder.

Reoperation after Failed Arthroscopic Treatment

Recent studies have shown that arthroscopic surgery may be advantageous in the treatment of small defects of OLTs, but favorable results have been less predictable for large and unstable osteochondral defects treated with the arthroscopic marrow-stimulation technique. Consequently, surgeons increasingly face the challenge of recommending a repeat surgical approach to second-line treatment. From the authors' ongoing study, they compared the clinical outcomes between repeated arthroscopic microfracture (n = 26) versus osteochondral autograft transplantation (OAT) (n = 22) in patients with a previous arthroscopic marrow-stimulation technique. An objective assessment showed no significant difference between the two groups at 6 months after the operations, but later follow-up showed significantly better evaluations in the OAT group. The repeat microfracture group showed significant deterioration over the 4.2-year follow-up ($P<.05$) but still had significant clinical improvement compared with the pretreatment evaluation. Based on the authors' preliminary research, they assumed that the primary treatment of OLTs should be arthroscopic and the OAT is reserve for failed previous surgery. Furthermore, the authors' results and those of other investigators using similar techniques may validate osteochondral transplantation as a viable alternative secondary procedure for treating unstable OLTs that are refractive to more commonly used surgical techniques. Large comparative studies with long-term follow-up providing a higher level of evidence are pending.

SUMMARY

The treatment of symptomatic OLTs has difficulties and limitations because of the poor regeneration of articular cartilage and the limited access to the ankle joint. It is important that the surgeon understand the causes of failure as well as the factors influencing the results of arthroscopic treatment of OLTs. The presence of such a risk factor may encourage surgeons to find new treatment strategies as well as counsel patients differently.

REFERENCES

1. Berndt AL, Harty M. Transchondral fractures (osteochondritis dissecans) of the talus. J Bone Joint Surg Am 1959;41:988–1020.
2. Baltzer AW, Arnold JP. Bone-cartilage transplantation from the ipsilateral knee for chondral lesions of the talus. Arthroscopy 2005;21(2):159–66.
3. König F. Über freie Körper in den Gelenken. Dtsch Z Chir 1888;27:90–109.
4. Schenck RC Jr, Goodnight JM. Osteochondritis dissecans. J Bone Joint Surg Am 1996;78(3):439–56.
5. Blevins FT, Steadman JR, Rodrigo JJ, et al. Treatment of articular cartilage defects in athletes: an analysis of functional outcome and lesion appearance. Orthopedics 1998;21(7):761–7 [discussion: 7–8].
6. Thordarson DB. Talar body fractures. Orthop Clin North Am 2001;32(1):65–77, viii.
7. Mullett H, Kennedy JG, Quinlan W. Subchondral talar cyst following open reduction and internal fixation of an ankle fracture. Foot Ankle Surg 1999;5(3):147–9.
8. Van Buecken K, Barrack RL, Alexander AH, et al. Arthroscopic treatment of transchondral talar dome fractures. Am J Sports Med 1989;17(3):350–5 [discussion: 5–6].
9. Anderson IF, Crichton KJ, Grattan-Smith T, et al. Osteochondral fractures of the dome of the talus. J Bone Joint Surg Am 1989;71(8):1143–52.
10. Pettine KA, Morrey BF. Osteochondral fractures of the talus. A long-term follow-up. J Bone Joint Surg Br 1987;69(1):89–92.
11. Pritsch M, Horoshovski H, Farine I. Arthroscopic treatment of osteochondral lesions of the talus. J Bone Joint Surg Am 1986;68(6):862–5.
12. Parisien JS. Arthroscopic treatment of osteochondral lesions of the talus. Am J Sports Med 1986;14(3):211–7.
13. Baker CL, Andrews JR, Ryan JB. Arthroscopic treatment of transchondral talar dome fractures. Arthroscopy 1986;2(2):82–7.
14. Flick AB, Gould N. Osteochondritis dissecans of the talus (transchondral fractures of the talus): review of the literature and new surgical approach for medial dome lesions. Foot Ankle 1985;5(4):165–85.
15. Frenkel SR, Di Cesare PE. Degradation and repair of articular cartilage. Front Biosci 1999;4:D671–85.
16. Easley ME, Scranton PE. Osteochondral autologous transfer system. Foot Ankle Clin 2003;8(2):275–90.
17. Zengerink M, Szerb I, Hangody L, et al. Current concepts: treatment of osteochondral ankle defects. Foot Ankle Clin 2006;11(2):331–59, vi.

18. van Dijk CN, Reilingh ML, Zengerink M, et al. Osteochondral defects in the ankle: why painful? Knee Surg Sports Traumatol Arthrosc 2010;18(5):570–80.
19. Choi WJ, Kim BS, Lee JW. Osteochondral lesion of the talus: could age be an indication for arthroscopic treatment? Am J Sports Med 2012;40(2):419–24.
20. Choi WJ, Park KK, Kim BS, et al. Osteochondral lesion of the talus: is there a critical defect size for poor outcome? Am J Sports Med 2009;37(10):1974–80.
21. Baker CL, Graham JM. Current concepts in ankle arthroscopy. Orthopedics 1993; 16(9):1027–35.
22. Giannini SS, Buda RR, Faldini CC, et al. Surgical treatment of osteochondral lesions of the talus in young active patients. J Bone Joint Surg Am 2005; 87(Suppl 2):28–41.
23. Gobbi A, Francisco RA, Lubowitz JH, et al. Osteochondral lesions of the talus: randomized controlled trial comparing chondroplasty, microfracture, and osteochondral autograft transplantation. Arthroscopy 2006;22(10):1085–92.
24. Kono M, Takao M, Naito K, et al. Retrograde drilling for osteochondral lesions of the talar dome. Am J Sports Med 2006;34(9):1450–6.
25. Savva N, Jabur M, Davies M, et al. Osteochondral lesions of the talus: results of repeat arthroscopic debridement. Foot Ankle Int 2007;28(6):669–73.
26. Alexander AH, Lichtman DM. Surgical treatment of transchondral talar-dome fractures (osteochondritis dissecans). Long-term follow-up. J Bone Joint Surg Am 1980;62(4):646–52.
27. Bryant DD, Siegel MG. Osteochondritis dissecans of the talus: a new technique for arthroscopic drilling. Arthroscopy 1993;9(2):238–41.
28. Shea MP, Manoli A. Osteochondral lesions of the talar dome. Foot Ankle 1993; 14(1):48–55.
29. Schuman L, Struijs PA, van Dijk CN. Arthroscopic treatment for osteochondral defects of the talus. Results at follow-up at 2 to 11 years. J Bone Joint Surg Br 2002;84(3):364–8.
30. Tol JL, Struijs PA, Bossuyt PM, et al. Treatment strategies in osteochondral defects of the talar dome: a systematic review. Foot Ankle Int 2000;21(2): 119–26.
31. Ferkel RD, Zanotti RM, Komenda GA, et al. Arthroscopic treatment of chronic osteochondral lesions of the talus: long-term results. Am J Sports Med 2008; 36(9):1750–62.
32. Baker CL Jr, Parisien JS. Arthroscopic surgery in osteocartilaginous lesions of the ankle. Operative arthroscopy. 2nd edition. Philadelphia: JB Lippincott; 1996. p. 1157–72.
33. Alford JW, Cole BJ. Cartilage restoration, part 1: basic science, historical perspective, patient evaluation, and treatment options. Am J Sports Med 2005; 33(2):295–306.
34. Furukawa T, Eyre DR, Koide S, et al. Biochemical studies on repair cartilage resurfacing experimental defects in the rabbit knee. J Bone Joint Surg Am 1980;62(1):79–89.
35. Nehrer S, Spector M, Minas T. Histologic analysis of tissue after failed cartilage repair procedures. Clin Orthop Relat Res 1999;(365):149–62.
36. Roden S, Tillegard P, Unanderscharin L. Osteochondritis dissecans and similar lesions of the talus: report of fifty-five cases with special reference to etiology and treatment. Acta Orthop Scand 1953;23(1):51–66.
37. Stone JW, Guhl JF. Ankle arthroscopy in the management of osteochondral lesions. In: Parisien JS, editor. Current Techniques in Arthroscopy. Philadelphia: Current Medicine; 1995. p. 226–37.

38. Ferkel RD, Scranton PE Jr, Stone JW, et al. Surgical treatment of osteochondral lesions of the talus. Instr Course Lect 2010;59:387–404.
39. Hunt SA, Sherman O. Arthroscopic treatment of osteochondral lesions of the talus with correlation of outcome scoring systems. Arthroscopy 2003;19(4): 360–7.
40. Robinson DE, Winson IG, Harries WJ, et al. Arthroscopic treatment of osteochondral lesions of the talus. J Bone Joint Surg Br 2003;85(7):989–93.
41. Chuckpaiwong B, Berkson EM, Theodore GH. Microfracture for osteochondral lesions of the ankle: outcome analysis and outcome predictors of 105 cases. Arthroscopy 2008;24(1):106–12.
42. Giannini S, Vannini F. Operative treatment of osteochondral lesions of the talar dome: current concepts review. Foot Ankle Int 2004;25(3):168–75.
43. Kreuz PC, Erggelet C, Steinwachs MR, et al. Is microfracture of chondral defects in the knee associated with different results in patients aged 40 years or younger? Arthroscopy 2006;22(11):1180–6.
44. Choi WJ, Lee JW, Han SH, et al. Chronic lateral ankle instability: the effect of intra-articular lesions on clinical outcome. Am J Sports Med 2008;36(11):2167–72.
45. Digiovanni BF, Fraga CJ, Cohen BE, et al. Associated injuries found in chronic lateral ankle instability. Foot Ankle Int 2000;21(10):809–15.
46. Han SH, Lee JW, Lee DY, et al. Radiographic changes and clinical results of osteochondral defects of the talus with and without subchondral cysts. Foot Ankle Int 2006;27(12):1109–14.
47. Hepple S, Winson IG, Glew D. Osteochondral lesions of the talus: a revised classification. Foot Ankle Int 1999;20(12):789–93.
48. Loomer R, Fisher C, Lloyd-Smith R, et al. Osteochondral lesions of the talus. Am J Sports Med 1993;21(1):13–9.
49. Ogilvie Harris DJ, Sarrosa EA. Arthroscopic treatment of post-traumatic cysts of the talus. Arthroscopy 2000;16(2):197–201.
50. Adams SB Jr, Viens NA, Easley ME, et al. Midterm results of osteochondral lesions of the talar shoulder treated with fresh osteochondral allograft transplantation. J Bone Joint Surg Am 2011;93(7):648–54.
51. Easley ME, Latt LD, Santangelo JR, et al. Osteochondral lesions of the talus. J Am Acad Orthop Surg 2010;18(10):616–30.
52. Gross AE, Agnidis Z, Hutchison CR. Osteochondral defects of the talus treated with fresh osteochondral allograft transplantation. Foot Ankle Int 2001;22(5): 385–91.
53. Cuttica DJ, Smith WB, Hyer CF, et al. Osteochondral lesions of the talus: predictors of clinical outcome. Foot Ankle Int 2011;32(11):1045–51.
54. Deol PB, Berlet GC, Hyer CF. Age stratification of outcomes for osteochondral lesions of the talus. Presented at American Orthopedic Foot and Ankle Society Summer Meeting. Vancouver, British Columbia, Canada July 15-18, 2009. [Epub ahead of print].
55. Knutsen G, Engebretsen L, Ludvigsen TC, et al. Autologous chondrocyte implantation compared with microfracture in the knee. A randomized trial. J Bone Joint Surg Am 2004;86(3):455–64.
56. Mithoefer K, Williams RJ, Warren RF, et al. The microfracture technique for the treatment of articular cartilage lesions in the knee. A prospective cohort study. J Bone Joint Surg Am 2005;87(9):1911–20.
57. Steadman JR, Briggs K, Rodrigo J, et al. Outcomes of microfracture for traumatic chondral defects of the knee: average 11-year follow-up. Arthroscopy 2003; 19(5):477–84.

58. Bergman RJ, Gazit D, Kahn AJ, et al. Age-related changes in osteogenic stem cells in mice. J Bone Miner Res 1996;11:568–77.
59. D'Ipplolito G, Schiller PC, Ricordi C, et al. Age-related osteogenic potential of mesenchymal stromal stem cells from human vertebral bone marrow. J Bone Miner Res 1999;14:1115–22.
60. Majors AK, Boehm CA, Nitto H, et al. Characterization of human bone marrow stromal cells with respect to osteoblastic differentiation. J Orthop Res 1997;15: 546–57.
61. Nishida S, Endo N, Yamagiwa H, et al. Number of osteoprogenitor cells in human bone marrow markedly decreases after skeletal maturation. J Bone Miner Metab 1999;17:171–7.
62. Brockbank KG, Ploemacher RE, van PC. An in vitro analysis of murine hemopoietic fibroblastoid progenitors and fibroblastoid cell function during aging. Mech Ageing Dev 1983;22:11–21.
63. Egrise D, Martin D, Vienne A, et al. The number of fibroblastic colonies formed from bone marrow is decreased and the in vitro proliferation rate of trabecular bone cells increased in aged rats. Bone 1992;13:355–61.
64. Oreffo RO, Bord S, Triffitt JT. Skeletal progenitor cells and ageing human populations. Clin Sci (Lond) 1998;94:549–55.
65. Christensen JC, Driscoll HL, Tencer AF. 1994 William J. Stickel Gold Award. Contact characteristics of the ankle joint. Part 2. The effects of talar dome cartilage defects. J Am Podiatr Med Assoc 1994;84(11):537–47.
66. Giannini S, Ceccarelli F, Girolami M, et al. Biological osteosynthesis in osteochondral lesions of the talus. Ital J Orthop Traumatol 1989;15(4):425–32.
67. Barth E, Hagen R. Juxta-articular bone cyst. Acta Orthop Scand 1982;53(2): 215–7.
68. Bauer TW, Dorfman HD. Intraosseous ganglion: a clinicopathologic study of 11 cases. Am J Surg Pathol 1982;6(3):207–13.
69. Kambolis C, Bullough PG, Jaffe HI. Ganglionic cystic defects of bone. J Bone Joint Surg Am 1973;55(3):496–505.
70. Mandelbaum BR, Browne JE, Fu F, et al. Articular cartilage lesions of the knee. Am J Sports Med 1998;26(6):853–61.
71. Marder RA, Hopkins G Jr, Timmerman LA. Arthroscopic microfracture of chondral defects of the knee: a comparison of two postoperative treatments. Arthroscopy 2005;21(2):152–8.
72. Schimmer RC, Dick W, Hintermann B. The role of ankle arthroscopy in the treatment strategies of osteochondritis dissecans lesions of the talus. Foot Ankle Int 2001;22(11):895–900.
73. Saxena A, Eakin C. Articular talar injuries in athletes: results of microfracture and autogenous bone graft. Am J Sports Med 2007;35(10):1680–7.

Particulated Juvenile Articular Cartilage Allograft Transplantation for Osteochondral Lesions of the Talus

Rebecca Cerrato, MD

KEYWORDS

- Particulated cartilage • DeNovo NT graft • Osteochondral lesion • Talus
- Restorative therapy

KEY POINTS

- Surgical strategies range from repair of cartilage through the formation of fibrocartilage (ie, reparative procedures) to a variety of restorative procedures, including tissue-engineering–based strategies.
- A novel treatment option involves the implantation of particulated articular cartilage obtained from a juvenile allograft donor, the DeNovo NT graft.
- This article reviews the DeNovo NT graft, its usage, and surgical technique.

HISTORICAL PERSPECTIVE

Surgical management of osteochondral lesions of the talus (OLTs) includes marrow stimulation techniques (drilling, microfracture, and abrasion arthroplasty) and a variety of restorative techniques. Marrow stimulation techniques, including microfracture, have long been considered first-line treatments for symptomatic OLTs because of their relative ease, ability to be performed arthroscopically, low expense, low morbidity, and quick recovery time. The microfracture technique results in fibrocartilage growth. The mechanical properties of fibrocartilage are less durable than hyaline cartilage.[1] Available literature suggests approximately 85% to 87% of patients report good to excellent results at follow-up.[2,3] Newer studies have started to further define the most appropriate OLTs for these techniques, noting that lesion size was the most important variable determining surgical success.[4,5]

Restorative techniques include osteochondral autograft transfer, fresh osteochondral allograft transplantation, and autologous chondrocyte implantation. The osteochondral autograft transfer system involves harvesting one or several (mosaicplasty)

Institute for Foot & Ankle Reconstruction, Mercy Medical Center, 301 St. Paul Place, Baltimore, MD 21202, USA
E-mail address: rcerrato@mdmercy.com

Foot Ankle Clin N Am 18 (2013) 79–87
http://dx.doi.org/10.1016/j.fcl.2012.12.005
1083-7515/13/$ – see front matter © 2013 Elsevier Inc. All rights reserved.

osteochondral plugs from a non–weight-bearing surface of a joint, typically the femoral condyles, supracondylar notch, or ipsilateral talus. This procedure allows the ability to transplant hyaline cartilage. Indications involve large lesions (>15 mm in diameter), cystic lesions, and failed OLTs treated previously with a marrow-stimulating technique. Numerous retrospective studies have reported good to excellent results in 91% to 100% of cases.[6] Gobbi and colleagues[7] reported on a prospective, nonrandomized trial comparing chondroplasty, microfracture, and osteochondral autograft. At a 2-year minimum follow-up, they found no significant difference in outcome scores among the 3 treatment groups. Concerns of this technique include technical difficulty, the typical requirement of a malleolar osteotomy to deliver the plug perpendicularly, and donor site morbidity, with incidence of knee pain reported in the literature ranging from 0% to 37%.[3]

Osteochondral allograft transplants are reserved for large, cystic, shoulder lesions, not amendable to other procedures. Structural grafts are used to reconstruct collapsed articular surfaces. These grafts are matched closely in size to the receipts and can be tailored to fit the extent of the defect. Several retrospective studies have reported good follow-up results, with one study at an average follow-up of 12 years[8] and the other study with a follow-up of 2 years.[9] Both studies included small numbers of 6 patients in each. Failures resulted in ankle arthrodeses. Disadvantages include donor tissue availability, disease transmission, and potential for immunologic reaction. Technically this is a demanding procedure, frequently requires an osteotomy during transplantation, and exact size matching can be variable.[2]

Autologous chondrocyte implantation (ACI) is a 2-stage procedure designed to regenerate tissue with a high percentage of hyalinelike cartilage, confirmed with histologic and immunohistochemical evaluations.[10] The first stage involves arthroscopic harvesting of chondrocytes, followed by cell culturing for approximately 6 weeks, concluded by a second surgery to transplant the cultured cells.[11] Newer-generation techniques, such as matrix-induced autologous chondrocyte implantation (MACI), deliver the cultured chondrocytes on a bioabsorbable collagen membrane. Indications include defects larger than 1 cm^2; unipolar, contained lesions; patients younger than 55 years; and previous failed surgical treatment of a symptomatic OLT. Disadvantages of this procedure include the requirement of 2 surgical procedures, frequent requirement of a malleolar osteotomy, and the technical difficultly of creating a sealed periosteal flap.[3] MACI and second-generation ACI techniques are not currently approved by the US Food and Drug Administration (FDA).

PARTICULATED JUVENILE CARTILAGE ALLOGRAFT TRANSPLANTATION

Minced, or particulated, articular cartilage graft is designed to create a hyalinelike cartilage within the defect, similar to ACI. The concept of using particulated cartilage tissue to repair cartilage defects was initially reported by Albrecht and colleagues[12] using a rabbit model. In recent years, an allograft preparation has become available as DeNovo Natural Tissue (NT) graft (Zimmer, Inc, Warsaw, IN; ISTO Technologies, St Louis, MO).[13] In the laboratory and in animal models, DeNovo NT grafts have demonstrated the ability of the transplanted cartilage cells to "escape" from the extracellular matrix, migrate, multiply, and form a new hyalinelike cartilage tissue matrix that integrates with the surrounding host tissue.[11,14] Cartilage fragments have been proposed as a valid source of cells in animal models, allowing coverage of large cartilage defects without requiring precultivation of cells.[15]

Articular cartilage undergoes structural, molecular, and mechanical changes with age. Deterioration of chondrocyte function accompanies these changes in the matrix, thus suggesting an age-related decline in the potential for cartilage repair. Because particulated juvenile cartilage allograft transplantation (PJCAT) is a preparation of immature articular cartilage, it has a much higher cellular density when compared with mature articular cartilage (**Fig. 1**).[16] Furthermore, juvenile chondrocytes have shown superior capabilities of producing cartilage extracellular matrix, sulfated glycosaminoglycans (s-GAG), which defines the cushioning properties of the tissue (**Fig. 2**).[17,18] Immature chondrocytes demonstrate greater mRNA levels for Type II and Type IX collagen.[17]

The first implantation of DeNovo NT graft was performed in May 2007 for a patella lesion.[19] Currently, applications to treat focal articular defects have expanded to the knee, talus, metatarsophalangeal joint, elbow, shoulder, and hip. In contrast to ACI, DeNovo NT graft is a single-stage procedure. Additional advantages for the use of PJCAT include that is there is no donor site morbidity, it is a technically simple procedure without the need for press-fit graphs, and, in most cases, a malleolar osteotomy is not required.[20,21] Disadvantages inherent to any allograft tissue include potential disease transmission and immunogenic reaction; however, there have been no reported complications or evidence of graft rejection to date. Additionally, tissue availability and cost must be considered when selecting this as an option.

DENOVO NT GRAFT

DeNovo NT graft is a cartilaginous tissue graft, obtained from juvenile allograft donors up to 13 years old, but typically younger than 2 years old. No stillborn or fetal tissue is used. Standard disease screening is performed on each tissue lot. It is provided as particulated tissue pieces each having a volume of approximately 1 mm^3. The tissue is packaged in a sterile primary package with a fortified salt solution and is stored at 19° to 26°C until ready to use. The maximum shelf life for each tissue lot is typically 35 days from the time the lot was released. Each package contains sufficient quantity to treat a 2.5-cm^2 defect. For defect areas larger than 2.5 cm^2, additional packages may be used. DeNovo NT graft is not recommended for lesions in excess of 5 cm^2. The FDA considers DeNovo NT as a minimally manipulated human tissue allograft, regulated similar to fresh osteochondral allografts and is available for use in clinical applications without an investigational device exemption.[22]

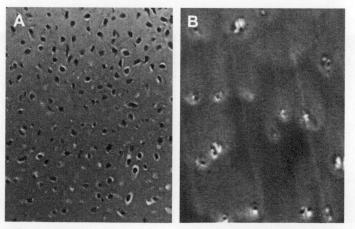

Fig. 1. Juvenile chondrocyte density (*A*) is approximately 8 to 10 times that of adult chondrocyte density (*B*).

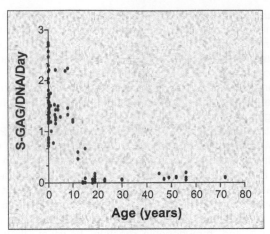

Fig. 2. Cartilage capacity to produce GAG decreases with age.

PREOPERATIVE PLANNING

Surgical management of symptomatic OLTs is considered in the patient who has failed conservative management.[23] Selecting the appropriate treatment strategy depends on several variables, including size of the lesion, contained versus uncontained defect, location of the talar lesion, surgeon experience, and history of previous surgical procedures.[3] Recommended indications for PJCAT include primary OLTs that are larger than 15 mm in diameter or patients who have failed a previous marrow-stimulating procedure. Specific contraindications include large cystic lesion or necrotic bone defects. Other contraindications include patients with an active infection at the surgical site, patients with clinically diagnosed autoimmune disease, diffuse ankle arthritis, or malalignment. Uncontained (shoulder) lesions are not excluded (**Fig. 3**). OLTs with small cystic bone lesions can be concomitantly treat with local bone grafting and application of DeNovo NT graft.

Appropriate imaging studies should be obtained for planning the number of lots required, possible need for an osteotomy, and requirement of autologous bone graft.

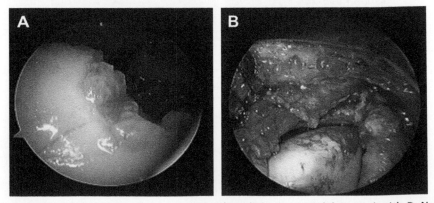

Fig. 3. Arthroscopic images of an uncontained medial talar OCD (*A*) treated with DeNovo NT graft (*B*).

Magnetic resonance imaging (MRI) of the talar lesion gives the most accurate dimension for the cartilage defect. Computed tomography scans can give an accurate footprint of the bone defect and the extent it may extend to the respective shoulder. Therefore, most patients with cystic OLTs obtain both imaging studies for preoperative evaluation.

SURGICAL TECHNIQUE

A standard ankle arthroscopy is routinely performed to evaluate the location and extent of the OLT, as well as address any associated pathology. Location of the lesion also can be evaluated with the ankle joint ranged to better determine the accessibility of the lesion through an arthrotomy versus malleolar osteotomy.[20] Initial debridement of the lesion can be performed through the scope or during the open portion of the procedure. Most surgical descriptions of this technique describe transplantation through an arthrotomy; however, many surgeons have started to perform the entire procedure through an all-arthroscopic technique.[10]

Arthroscopic Transplantation

Following the arthroscopic debridement of the lesion, the joint is thoroughly dried using an abdominal insufflator at 20 mm Hg in one portal and a Frazier suction tip attached to suction in the other portal. The joint is allowed to dry for several minutes, placing the suction tip at the base of the debrided lesion. Eye spears are introduced through either portal to further dry the subchondral base. An initial thin layer of fibrin glue is delivered onto the base of the OLT through a preloaded syringe.

The DeNovo graft pieces are loaded into a 10-gauge angiocatheter and delivered to the lesion through the arthroscopic portal, with the insufflations discontinued. The graft particles are arranged to cover the entire OLT using an arthroscopic probe or Freer elevator. A second layer of fibrin glue is applied over the graft and the abdominal insufflator is restarted to maintain a dry joint space, until the fibrin glue is firm to touch. The arthroscopic equipment is withdrawn and the portals are closed using standard technique.

Open (Arthrotomy) Transplantation

Following the arthroscopic portion, a medial or lateral arthrotomy is performed, incorporating the arthroscopy portal into the skin incision. The foot is plantarflexed and visualization of the OLT is performed. It is not necessary to have perpendicular access to the lesion; however, the entire lesion should be accessible for preparation and transplantation. If the entire lesion is not visualized, either a tibial plafondplasty is used or the joint is distracted with a large Hintermann distractor. Adams and colleagues[20] described using a curved one-quarter-inch osteotome to remove a portion of the anterior tibial plafond. They cautioned not to remove more than 1 cm of the nonarticular tibia in any dimension. Smaller plafondplasties are not repaired, whereas those approaching 1 cm can be secured using small-fragmentary screw or bioabsorbable pin fixation. Malleolar osteotomies are typically unnecessary; however, posterior and uncontained lesions that extend far into its respective gutter can be difficult to visualize with a plafondplasty, therefore preoperative planning and counseling are necessary.

Arthroscopic curettes and beaver blades are used to debride the lesion, creating stable, vertical walls, and a well-defined base. The joint should be thoroughly irrigated and dried. A thigh tourniquet is used. The dimension of the lesion is created by pressing a thin piece of sterile aluminum foil into the defect, creating a template. On the sterile field, stage together the DeNovo NT graft package and fibrin preparation. The fibrin preparation should be placed in a double-barrel syringe and warmed to room temperature. The foil lid on the DeNovo graft package is carefully peeled and the preservation medium is aspirated using a 25-gauge needle. A Freer elevator is useful for delivering the cartilage pieces to the foil mold, arranging them evenly across the base of the mold. The fibrin glue preparation is gently applied to the mold to embed the particulated pieces to fill three-fourths of the mold depth. The graft should not sit proud, similar to an osteochondral plug. The mold is typically allowed to set for 5 to 10 minutes. Once the graft is firm, the foil edges are pulled to straighten the foil (**Fig. 4**). A thin layer of fibrin glue is applied to the base of the defect. The graft is then carefully manipulated into the defect and fibrin glue is used to seal the edges of the graft.

Alternately, the molding of the aluminum foil can present a challenge at the talus because of exposure and often the lesion is grafted without using the foil. Once the base of the defect has a thin layer of fibrin glue, a Freer elevator can be used to directly transfer the particulated pieces onto the defect again in a uniform, single layer (**Fig. 5**). Once the lesion is adequately covered by the cartilage, a second application of fibrin glue is applied and allowed to set for a similar amount of time. From here, the ankle is dorsiflexed until the lesion is covered and axial compression is applied to mold the graft using the contour of the tibial articular surface. This is typically held for several minutes. Incisions are closed in a standard fashion. A well-padded splint is applied with the ankle in neutral flexion and the patient is kept non–weight bearing.

POSTOPERATIVE MANAGEMENT

The patient returns 10 to 14 days following surgery. Sutures are removed, and the patient is placed in a removable boot. The patient remains non–weight bearing for 4 to 6 weeks, starting ankle range-of-motion exercises once the boot is applied.[20,21]

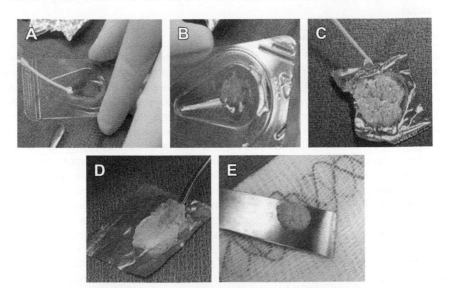

Fig. 4. Preparation of the DeNovo NT graft (*A, B*), placement of particulated cartilage into foil mold with fibrin glue (*C*), and delivery of form cartilage graft (*D, E*).

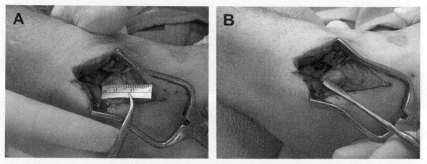

Fig. 5. An anterolateral OLT after debridement (*A*) and following graft transplantation (*B*).

After 6 weeks, the patient progresses to full weight bearing and discontinues the boot as tolerated. Physical therapy is initiated typically at 6 weeks. The rehabilitation program focuses initially on protection of the cartilage repair process and then progresses toward controlled loading, increased range of motion, and progressive muscle strengthening. Low-impact activities are typically started at 4 months.

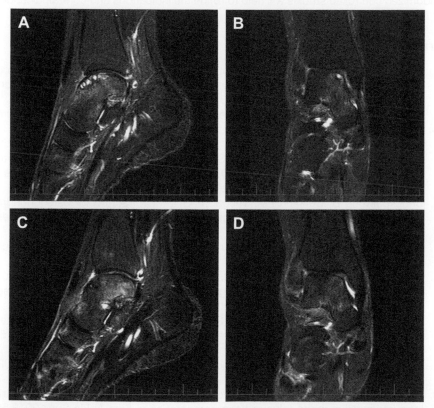

Fig. 6. Preoperative sagittal (*A*) and coronal (*B*) MRI images of a 24-year-old woman with a symptomatic, large medial OLT. Postoperative sagittal (*C*) and coronal (*D*) MRI images of the same patient 1 year following treatment with calcaneal bone graft to the cystic bone defects and DeNovo NT graft transplant.

RESULTS

To date, there are only 2 clinical studies on the use of DeNovo NT for symptomatic cartilage lesions in the knee and no published results on its use for the treatment of OLTs.[19,22] The first is a case report on the use of particulated juvenile cartilage tissue in the treatment of a patella cartilage defect.[19] At 2-year follow-up, the patient reported improvement in both pain and function. MRI evaluation demonstrated resolution of preoperative bony edema. Similar findings have been confirmed with 1-year follow-up MRI images on patients treated for OLTs with DeNovo NT grafts (**Fig. 6**). The second is a multicenter, prospective, single-arm study of 25 patients with femoral condyle or trochlea OCDs. Four patients had completed 24-month follow-up at the time of the report, with consistent improvement in outcome scores.[22] Several retrospective and prospective studies are ongoing to determine the use and efficacy of this treatment approach in patients with symptomatic OLTs.

SUMMARY

The transplantation of particulated, juvenile cartilage tissue allograft appears to be a promising new treatment option for the patient with symptomatic OLT. Further study is needed before evidence-based recommendations can be made. Prospective randomized controlled studies will help to refine the indications and contraindications for DeNovo NT.

REFERENCES

1. LaPrade RF, Bursch LS, Olson EJ, et al. Histologic and immunohistochemical characteristics of failed articular cartilage resurfacing procedures for osteochondritis of the knee: a case series. Am J Sports Med 2008;36:360–8.
2. Ferkel RD, Scranton PE, Stone JW, et al. Surgical treatment of osteochondral lesions of the talus. Instr Course Lect 2010;59:387–404.
3. Zengerink M, Struijs PA, Tol JL, et al. Treatment of osteochondral lesions of the talus: a systematic review. Knee Surg Sports Traumatol Arthrosc 2010;18:238–46.
4. Choi WJ, Park KK, Kim BS, et al. Osteochondral lesion of the talus: is there a critical defect size for poor outcome? Am J Sports Med 2009;37:1974–80.
5. Chuckpaiwong B, Berkson EM, Theodore GH. Microfracture for osteochondral lesion of the ankle: outcome analysis and outcome predictors of 105 cases. Arthroscopy 2008;24:106–12.
6. McHale P, Pinney. Current concepts review: osteochondral lesions of the talus. Foot Ankle Int 2010;31(1):90–101.
7. Gobbi A, Francisco RA, Lubowitz JH, et al. Osteochondral lesions of the talus: randomized controlled trial comparing chondroplasty, microfracture, and osteochondral autograft transplantation. Arthroscopy 2006;22:1085–92.
8. Gross AE, Agnidis Z, Hutchison CR. Osteochondral defects of the talus treated with fresh osteochondral allograft transplantation. Foot Ankle Int 2001;22(5): 385–91.
9. Raikin SM. Stage IV: massive osteochondral defects of the talus. Foot Ankle Clin 2004;9(4):737–44.
10. Kruse DL, Ng A, Paden M, et al. Arthroscopic DeNovo NT juvenile allograft cartilage implantation in the talus: a case presentation. J Foot Ankle Surg 2012;51: 218–21.
11. Ahmed T, Hincke MT. Strategies for articular cartilage lesion repair and functional restoration. Tissue Eng 2010;16(3):305–29.

12. Albrecht F, Roessner A, Zimmermann E. Closure of osteochondral lesions using chondral fragments and fibrin adhesive. Arch Orthop Trauma Surg 1983;101: 213–7.
13. McCormick F, Yanke A, Provencher MT, et al. Minced articular cartilage-basic science, surgical technique, and clinical application. Sports Med Arthrosc 2008;16:217–20.
14. Farr J, Cole BJ, Sherman S, et al. Particulated articular cartilage: CAIS and DeNovo NT. J Knee Surg 2012;25(1):23–9.
15. Bonasia DE, Martin JA, Marmotti A, et al. Cocultures of adult and juvenile chondrocytes compared with adult and juvenile chondral fragments. In vitro matrix production. Am J Sports Med 2011;20(10):1–7.
16. McNickle AG, Provencher MT, Cole BJ. Overview of existing cartilage repair technology. Sports Med Arthrosc 2008;16:196–201.
17. Adkisson HD, Martin JA, Amendola RL, et al. The potential of human allogeneic juvenile chondrocytes for restoration of articular cartilage. Am J Sports Med 2010; 38:1324–33.
18. Feder J, Adkisson HD, Kizer N, et al. The promise of chondral repair using neo-cartilage. In: Sandell LJ, Grodzinsky AJ, editors. Tissue engineering in musculo-skeletal clinical practices. Rosemont (IL): AAOS Pub; 2004. p. 219–26.
19. Bonner KF, Daner W, Yao JQ. 2-year postoperative evaluation of a patient with a symptomatic full-thickness patellar cartilage defect repaired with particulated juvenile cartilage tissue. J Knee Surg 2010;23:109–14.
20. Adams SB, Yao JQ, Schon LC. Particulated juvenile articular cartilage allograft transplantation for osteochondral lesions of the talus. Tech Foot Ankle Surg 2011;10(2):92–8.
21. Hatic S, Berlet G. Particulated juvenile articular cartilage graft (DeNovo NT Graft) for treatment of osteochondral lesions of the talus. Foot Ankle Spec 2010;3(6): 361–4.
22. Farr J, Yao JQ. Chondral defect repair with particulated juvenile cartilage allograft. Cartilage 2011;2(4):346–53.
23. Mitchell ME, Giza E, Sullivan MR. Cartilage transplantation techniques for talar cartilage lesions. J Am Acad Orthop Surg 2009;17:407–14.

Why Allograft Reconstruction for Osteochondral Lesion of the Talus? The Osteochondral Autograft Transfer System Seemed to Work Quite Well

Anish R. Kadakia, MD[a],*, Norman Espinosa, MD[b]

KEYWORDS

- Osteochondral lesion of the talus • Allograft reconstruction
- Osteochondral autograft transfer system • Revision surgery

KEY POINTS

- Both autograft and allograft reconstruction have documented success in the treatment of osteochondral defects of the talus.
- Universal availability and known chondrocyte viability makes autograft OATS an excellent option for recurrent, deep (>5 mm), or moderate-sized (<2 cm^2) defects.
- Allograft reconstruction is best suited for defects with a large diameter, large cystic component, or heavily involving the shoulder of the talus.
- Understanding and communicating the unique risks of each treatment to the patient is critical when making the choice for reconstruction.

INTRODUCTION

Osteochondral lesions of the talus (OCLT) are a challenging pathologic entity despite the advancements that have been made to treat focal deficits of articular cartilage. This entity was first described in the talus as an osteochondritis dissecans by Kappis[1] in 1922, who noted an association with traumatic injury. Given the lack of an inflammatory component to the lesion, the term osteochondral lesion of the talus is more appropriate. The first classification system was devised by Berndt and Harty[2] in 1959 and, despite numerous other classifications that have been created since, it is still widely used. The utility of the multiple classification systems with regard to the most

[a] Department of Orthopedic Surgery, Northwestern University – Feinberg School of Medicine, Suite 1350, 676 North St Clair Street, Chicago, IL 60611, USA; [b] Department of Orthopaedics, University of Zurich, Balgrist, Forchstrasse 340, Zürich 8008, Switzerland
* Corresponding author.
E-mail address: Kadak259@gmail.com

Foot Ankle Clin N Am 18 (2013) 89–112
http://dx.doi.org/10.1016/j.fcl.2012.12.006
1083-7515/13/$ – see front matter © 2013 Elsevier Inc. All rights reserved.

foot.theclinics.com

appropriate treatment is limited. The addition of a Stage V by Scranton and McDermott[3] in 2001, describing a subchondral cyst with an intact cartilage cap, does indicate that retrograde drilling in the lesion may be indicated, avoiding disruption of the articular surface (**Fig. 1**). Raikin[4] proposed a Stage VI lesion defined by volumes of greater than 3000 mm,[3] which could be treated with allograft reconstruction. However, this leaves a large portion of lesions for which no specific treatment regimen can be recommended based on classification. The efficacy and determination of the most appropriate graft reconstruction, that is, allograft reconstruction versus the osteochondral autograft transfer system (OATS), constitute the focus of this review. To maintain a clear distinction between autograft and allograft reconstruction, in this article the term OATS refers to autograft reconstruction of the talus.

The use of arthroscopic debridement with concomitant microfracture or drilling is a very effective initial treatment, with good to excellent results reported in 70% to 90% of the patients.[5–9] Determining the need for cartilage replacement treatment on the diameter of the lesion has been advocated, but is not universally supported by the literature. Chuckpaiwong and colleagues[9] reviewed results of arthroscopy and microfracture in 105 patients and noted that for lesions larger than 1.5 cm^2, only 1 patient met the criteria for success, compared with success in all patients with smaller lesions. The 1.5-cm^2 limit for a successful treatment with microfracture was reinforced in a review of 120 patients correlating poor outcome in 80% of patients with lesions larger than 1.5 cm^2 on magnetic resonance imaging (MRI).[10] Although depth of the lesion was not evaluated as an independent variable, lesions that are larger than 1.5 cm^2 without loss of the subchondral bone may be more amenable to

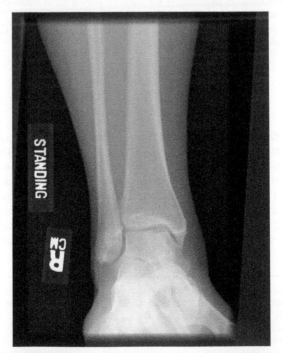

Fig. 1. Plain mortise radiograph of a Stage V lesion in a patient with a symptomatic OCLT with radiographic evidence of a cystic defect that demonstrated an intact cartilage cap after diagnostic arthroscopy.

arthroscopy and microfracture than those with a bony defect. In a prospective non-randomized study evaluating the effect of chondroplasty, microfracture, and OATS treatment, no significant difference in outcome was noted at 2-year follow-up despite the mean lesion size being 4.5 cm^2 in the microfracture group and 4 cm^2 in the chondroplasty group.[11] However, when evaluating results with respect to size of the lesion, both OATS and microfracture treatment showed an increasingly poor outcome correlated with an increase in the size of the defect.[11] Inability to recreate the exact anatomy of talus, restore 100% of the cartilage surface, and possible preexisting alteration to the tibial articular cartilage may account for the increasingly poor outcomes in larger lesions despite the use of an OATS technique.

Cartilage transplantation techniques for revision surgery would seem to be a straight-forward indication; however, this is not the case. A study by Savva and colleagues[12] determined that good to excellent results can be achieved in 82% of patients with repeat arthroscopic debridement and microfracture. In their series, patients with a cystic lesion were excluded and all patients had lesions that were smaller than 1.5 cm^2. Schuman and colleagues[8] evaluated 16 patients who underwent revision debridement and drilling after a failed prior intervention that consisted of either debridement or drilling, but not a combination of the 2 techniques. The investigators noted a 75% good to excellent result in this population after a minimum of 2 years of follow-up. However, neither size nor depth of the lesion was reported. Given the limited data, revision arthroscopy may be appropriate for small lesions less than 1.5 cm^2 and those that do not have a cystic component. The literature does not support revision arthroscopy for larger lesions or those that have a cavitary defect.

Despite the lack of objective evidence to determine the need for an autograft or allograft osteochondral reconstruction of the talus, some indications for their use can still be determined.

- Lesions with loss of cartilage continuity and a cystic defect or depth of greater than 5 mm may benefit from a bone/cartilage transplant procedure (**Fig. 2**). The primary benefit over isolated cartilage transplantation is the ability to concomitantly reconstruct the bony defect, restoring the anatomy of the talus. Concomitant cancellous bone grafting of the lesion with placement of autologous chondrocytes (autologous chondrocyte implantation or matrix-assisted autologous chondrocyte implantation) or allograft cartilage on top of the graft is an alternative; however, limited data are available with which to evaluate the efficacy of these techniques in the setting of a bony defect.

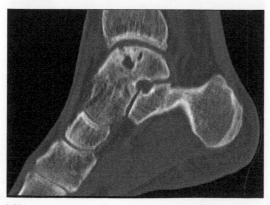

Fig. 2. CT scan of a different patient with multiple cystic defects greater than 5 mm in depth.

- Large-volume defects of greater than 3 cm^3 as proposed by Raikin clearly need a form of reconstruction that is amenable only to allograft reconstruction.
- In cases of repeatedly failed arthroscopic treatment, cartilage transplantation would be appropriate regardless of the size of the lesion.
- The authors also consider graft reconstruction in cases of failed arthroscopic treatment in lesions larger than 1.5 cm^2 given the correlation of poor outcomes in this patient population (**Fig. 3**).

OSTEOCHONDRAL AUTOLOGOUS TRANSPLANTATION

Wagner[13] was first to introduce the concept of cartilage-bone–cylinder transplantation to treat osteochondrosis dissecans of the knee. During the last 3 decades, and as an alternative to allograft transplantation, OATS has become an appealing solution to treat medium to large-sized osteochondral lesions of the talus. In contrast to other surgical treatments, which address the cartilage (autologous chondrocyte transplantation), bone (eg, retrograde drilling) or both (debridement, curettage, and drilling), an OATS provides an osteochondral unit with viable cells, which serves to replace the entire lesion.

Benefits of Autograft

- As an autograft is used, there is no risk of transmitting diseases (eg, human immunodeficiency virus or hepatitis C).
- There is no risk of transplant rejection, and the longevity of the cartilaginous cells is higher than that for allogenic material.[14]
- Ankle cartilage is less responsive to catabolic stimulation and is thus less susceptible to damage.
- In addition, when compared with other procedures (eg, autologous chondrocyte implantation), it demonstrates a reasonable cost-effectiveness.

Limitations of Autograft

- Donor-site morbidity in the knee including persistent pain, difficult kneeling, and patellar instability can occur.

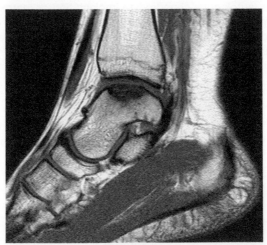

Fig. 3. Sagittal MR image demonstrating a moderate-sized lesion greater than 1.5 cm^2 that is an appropriate candidate for graft reconstruction, especially if a prior arthroscopic procedure has failed.

- The amount of autologous material is limited. Therefore, larger defects still pose a problem. Using an OATS technique to treat a massive talar lesion requires many graft cylinders to be taken, resulting in greater donor-site morbidity for the patient.
- Inability to reconstruct the shoulder lesions of the talus.
- The thickness of knee cartilage is 2 to 3 times greater than that of the ankle but is less stiff and more susceptible to damage.

Indications and Contraindications

As stated previously, there is no definitive indication for the procedure.

- Lesions with loss of cartilage continuity and a cystic defect or depth of greater than 5 mm, failed prior arthroscopic management of large (>1.5 cm) lesions, or repeatedly failed arthroscopic treatment regardless of size are all excellent indications.
- Patients with evidence also of tibial cartilage degeneration are not appropriate candidates.
- In defects that are 2 to 3 cm in diameter, the use of an autograft may be associated with excessive morbidity to the knee, and allografting should be considered.
- Lesions greater than 3 cm in diameter require allograft reconstruction given the significant amount of graft required.
- Preoperative sizing of the lesion can be performed by computed tomography (CT) scan (superior for bony defects) or MRI scan; however, intraoperative measurement after debridement is the most accurate measurement. Familiarity with the mosaicplasty technique is critical, for instance in the setting of a larger defect than anticipated, as a single plug may not correct the defect when performing an OATS.

Sites for Graft Harvest

The most common site for graft harvest is the ipsilateral knee, conferring the advantage that it is a true autograft. The same applies for autografts taken from the ipsilateral talus. The latter provides only small amounts of graft but avoids violation of a normal joint (ie, the knee).

Surgical Technique

Different approaches are used to treat medial or lateral osteochondral lesions of the talus.

Medial osteochondral lesions of the talus

The approach is dependent on the site of the lesions. Anteromedial lesions can be approached through an anteromedial route with a concomitant plafondplasty. This approach should allow adequate exposure for the anterior half of the talus and eliminates the morbidity from an osteotomy. Lesions that are in the central and posterior aspect of the talus are best visualized with an osteotomy. A recent cadaveric study demonstrated that plafondplasty with plantarflexion of the talus allows visualization of the anterior 75% of the talar dome.[15] However, the plafondplasty was aggressive as discussed by the investigators, and the ability to perform a reconstruction was not determined. Therefore, caution should be exercised in attempting to reconstruct central and posterior lesions without an osteotomy.

To perform the osteotomy, a medial skin incision of approximately 10 cm is performed midway over the malleolus. The subcutaneous tissue is split, and the saphenous nerve and vein mobilized anteriorly. Posteriorly, the flexor retinaculum is identified and the sheath of the posterior tibial tendon is opened. A Hohmann retractor is inserted in such a fashion as to protect the flexor tendons and neurovascular bundle. Another Hohmann retractor is inserted into the medial corner of the ankle joint. Before starting with the osteotomy, the drill holes for later fixation are prepared (2.5- and 3.5-mm drill bits). A K-wire is inserted, which should traject the tibial plafond at the lateral extent of osteochondral lesion (as seen on intraoperative fluoroscopy). By means of an oscillating saw the osteotomy is done until the subchondral zone is reached, and is completed using an osteotome. The medial malleolus is reflected and the talus accessed (**Fig. 4**). After having transferred the osteochondral plugs, the medial malleolus is reduced and fixed by means of 2 3.5-mm screws. Placement of a transverse screw from medial to lateral minimizes the risk of superior translation of the osteotomy (**Fig. 5**).

Lateral osteochondral lesions of the talus
In general, to access and expose the anterior and midportion of the lateral talus, the anterior talofibular ligament can be detached and the talus subluxed anteriorly. Usually most of the lateral osteochondral lesions can be approached by an anterolateral arthrotomy with or without detachment of the anterior talofibular ligament, without the need for dissection of the inferior tibiofibular ligament. In their series of Type V lesions, Scranton and McDermott[3] did not require any lateral osteotomies for exposure of the lateral talus.

As with medial lesions, an anterolateral exposure combined with or without a plafondplasty allows access the anterior half of the lateral talus. More central and posterior lesions may require an osteotomy. A lateral skin incision over the fibula and anterior to its tip is performed. The length measures approximately 10 to 13 cm and can be increased as desired. Care is taken not to injure the superficial peroneal nerve. The inferior extensor retinaculum needs to be opened, and tendons of the musculus extensor digitorum brevis are pulled medially while the perforating branch of the fibular artery is preserved. Some investigators recommend a V-shaped fibular osteotomy, whereas others perform a simple osteotomy of the lateral malleolus. A V-shaped fibular osteotomy provides intrinsic stability and prevents secondary dislocation during and after fixation. Alternatively, to access the talar dome, removal of the anterior tibial plafond has been described.[16] However, osteochondral lesions often are found in the posterior part of the talus, making this kind of approach impractical. In

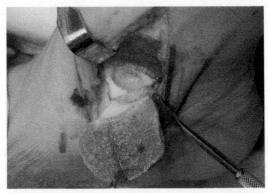

Fig. 4. Reflection of the medial malleolus allows visualization of the osteochondral defect. For lesions that extend slightly more central, the osteotomy can be allowed to exit more laterally; however, this will cause disruption of the weight-bearing articular surface as was done in this case.

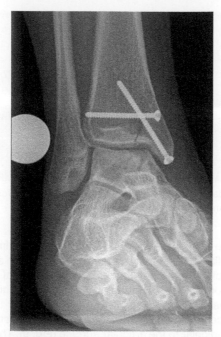

Fig. 5. Final fixation of the medial malleolar osteotomy was performed with the use of a transverse screw to prevent proximal migration. The width of the saw blade will result in bone loss, and this may result in superior translation of the fragment with compression from the oblique screw.

addition, removal of the anterior tibial plafond could weaken the tibial plafond and medial malleolus. Sammarco and Makwana[17] adopted this method but used only a small osteochondral window (10 mm wide, 20 mm deep, 30 mm in height), which was placed directly over the osteochondral lesion of the talus.

Several other articles have reported on different types of osteotomies of the fibula or of the fibula and Chaput fragment used to approach extensive lateral talar lesions. Gautier and colleagues[18] performed a fibula and Chaput fragment osteotomy, whereas Draper and Fallat[19] described an oblique osteotomy distal to the syndesmosis. Tochigi and colleagues[20] introduced the technique of an anterolateral tibial osteotomy and pointed out that fibular osteotomy can be complicated by malunion or insufficiency of the syndesmosis. Compared with a simple osteotomy of the anterolateral corner, it is also a more extensive procedure.

The ankle is held in supination and plantarflexion to expose the talar dome. At this point the defect can be addressed. After plug transfer, the fibula is reduced and secured by means of screws or a plate.

Harvest and transfer of osteochondral grafts
Once the ankle is opened, the osteochondral lesion can be accessed. The osteochondral lesion is debrided sharply until reaching a stable circumferential rim. A sizing guide is used on the talar site to measure the size of the defect. Using a recipient-site chisel, which is held perpendicular to the lesion, osteochondral plugs of 10 to 15 mm depth are removed (**Fig. 6**). The chisel is turned 90° and then 90° again, and the osteochondral cylinder extracted. Another tamp is used impact the cancellous bone and to measure the new depth of the future plug (**Fig. 7**).

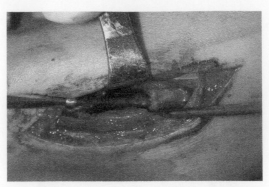

Fig. 6. Removal of the damaged articular surface and bone is performed with a cylindrical chisel. (*Courtesy of* Dr Anand Vora, Chicago, IL.)

On the femoral site a mini-arthrotomy is performed (approximately 5-cm skin incision lateral to the patella and proximal to the knee joint line) to access the knee joint. The soft tissues are split and the patella held onto the medial side. Now the lateral femoral condyle is exposed (**Fig. 8**). By means of a donor-site chisel the osteochondral plug is harvested. Usually the donor-site chisel is 1 mm wider than the recipient-site chisel. In so doing the contour of the surface and the radius must be taken into consideration, staying perpendicular to the articular surface (**Fig. 9**). The length of the plug is measured, and at times needs trimming. Once the correct length is achieved, the plug is inserted into the talar bone. The plug should be placed flush to the native cartilage to allow for appropriate load sharing of the transplanted cartilage (**Fig. 10**). If the plug is not placed flush with the talar surface, the superficial hyaline cartilage layer could be sheared off and damaged.

Use of a single large plug to fill the defect maximizes the amount of hyaline cartilage restoration which, however, may be associated with increased donor-site morbidity.[21,22] The use of multiple smaller plugs (3.5–6.5 mm) may decrease this risk and additionally allows for superior matching of the talar contour. However, mosaicplasty is associated with increased reparative fibrocartilage secondary to the gaps between each plug, and

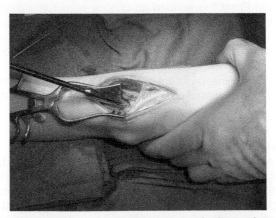

Fig. 7. A tamp is used to compress the cancellous bone to facilitate placement of the donor osteochondral plug, and allows accurate measurement of the correct depth. (*Courtesy of* Dr Anand Vora, Chicago, IL.)

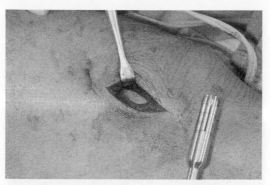

Fig. 8. Mini-arthrotomy is performed to expose the lateral femoral condyle. The skin incision typically does not require more than 5 cm length. (*Courtesy of* Dr Anand Vora, Chicago, IL.)

the degeneration of fibrocartilage of up to one-third of the total surface area of the graft secondary to trauma during harvest and implantation.[23–25]

Postoperative Management

For the first 2 days after surgery the foot is placed in a splint and elevated to reduce swelling. Two weeks postoperatively, the splint is removed and the patient is placed into a removable CAM walker. Gentle passive range of motion in the ankle is now encouraged to maintain movement and cartilage nutrition. The patient is kept non–weight-bearing for 6 weeks. Fifty percent weight-bearing in the CAM walker may be initiated after 6 weeks and continued for a further 2 weeks. Full weight-bearing should be achieved by 8 weeks postoperatively. Physical therapy including strengthening exercises is begun at 8 weeks postoperatively, with transition to full weight-bearing exercises at 10 weeks with the use a lace-up brace.

Pitfalls

- The malleolar osteotomy should have perfect anatomic congruency at the end of the procedure. No intra-articular step-off should be seen at the end of the procedure. To do so, a transversal lag screw is inserted from medial to lateral, followed by an oblique screw.

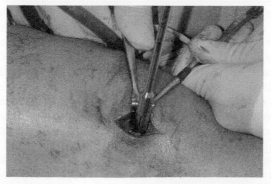

Fig. 9. Matched donor-site chisel is used to harvest the graft. Care must be taken to stay perpendicular to the articular surface to obtain an appropriately shaped plug. (*Courtesy of* Dr Anand Vora, Chicago, IL.)

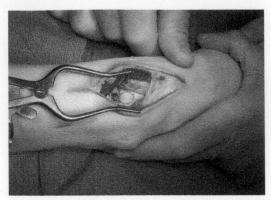

Fig. 10. Final appearance of the graft. Note that the plug is flush with the native articular cartilage. Exposure was facilitated with the use of a limited plafondplasty in this case. (*Courtesy of* Dr Anand Vora, Chicago, IL.)

- The graft must not be longer than the recipient site. Thus it is important to measure graft height and recipient-site depth properly. Impacting the graft to force it into the recipient site could possibly lead to delamination of the hyaline cartilage layer and thus destroy the graft.
- The chisels should be oriented perpendicular to the recipient-donor sites as well, to create even surfaces of the osteochondral plugs.
- At times a graft can be incongruent and, therefore, cause postoperative pain and early failure. In such a case the graft should be put back into the donor site and a new and more congruent graft harvested.
- Malposition of graft: Use the "corkscrew" instrument to adjust the graft plug. The instrument should not be driven through the cartilage layer, so as to prevent any damage to the layer.
- Avoid any graft harvest site fracturing into an adjacent harvest site; this might be a danger when harvesting multiple osteochondral plugs.
- On the recipient site, overlapping areas may be created (intersecting circles) in order to stuff the lesion zone with osteochondral plugs.

Complications

Complications are not frequently reported in the literature. Infections and wound-healing problems range from 0.4% to 5%.[26–29] Failure of graft incorporation has been reported, but it is very difficult to obtain an accurate percentage. This inaccuracy may be secondary to the fact that detection by means of MRI and CT is difficult and not routinely done in most of the reviewed study designs used for this article. Donor-site morbidity ranges between 15% and 50%.[27,30–33] More recently, in a large study with 112 patients, Paul and collegues[32] concluded that harvesting the graft from the ipsilateral knee can potentially lead to functional impairment, and that surgeons should be aware of the potentially negative effect of a higher body mass index on clinical outcomes after surgery. However, the functional outcome of the knee was not affected by the number and size of grafts nor the age of patients.

Other possible complications include malleolar nonunion, degenerative changes in the long term, and persisting pain despite radiographic evidence of full incorporation. Temporary femoropatellar pain has been reported in 10% of cases.[14]

Results

In 1997, Hangody and coworkers[30] reported on their results of mosaicplasty in 11 patients. All patients were reviewed after a follow-up of 12 to 28 months with an average follow-up of 16 months. All patients were evaluated using the Bandi clinical scoring system and the Hannover score, both of which improved. Three patients showed occasional knee pain, 1 had pain with activity, and 1 revealed an extension lag of 10° at the knee joint. With regard to the operated ankle, all patients had an excellent result. Shortly after, the same authors published the results of 36 consecutive patients who had been treated between 1992 and 1997 and followed up for 2 to 7 years after initial surgery.[34] All patients achieved full range of motion and none of the grafts showed subsidence. According to the Hannover scores, 28 patients rated their ankles as excellent, 6 as good, and 2 as moderate.

Baltzer and Arnold[35] were able to demonstrate the effectiveness of OATS in 43 patients. Of note, during the first postoperative year the range of motion at the ankle improved.

Al-Shaikh[36] and colleagues presented their results of OATS used in 19 patients. The average age of their group was 32 years, comparable with previously published works. All patients had failed nonoperative treatment and 13 patients had undergone some form of surgery before OATS. After an average follow-up of 15 months, the final American Orthopedic Foot and Ankle Society (AOFAS) score averaged 88 points (maximum 100 points). Although occasional pain was noted in most patients, all showed an excellent function, range of motion, stability, and hindfoot alignment. Assessment of the knee was done using the Lysholm knee score, the average value of which was 97 points (maximum 100 points).

Another study by Valderrabano and colleagues[31] reviewed 12 patients, 92% of whom reported good to excellent satisfaction and 8% poor satisfaction. The visual analog scale (VAS) of pain, the AOFAS, the sports activity scores, and the ankle function improved significantly. However, almost 50% of patients reported donor-site morbidity at the knee joint at 72 months' follow-up. In 10 of 10 ankles a recurrent lesion was found, and only 4 patients (33%) reached their preinjury level of sport.

Sammarco and Makwana[17] studied the results of 12 patients who had been treated by means of OATS using autografts harvested from the ipsilateral medial or lateral talar articular facet. The average age of the patients was 41 years and the duration of symptoms 90 months. Significant improvement regarding AOFAS scores was found (from 64 points preoperatively to 91 points postoperatively) after a mean follow-up time of 25 months. The investigators found that the younger the patient and the less arthritic changes preexisting, the better the outcome. No complications were found at the donor site.

Schottle and colleagues[14] presented their results after OATS procedure in the treatment of medium-sized osteochondral lesions of the talus. Thirty-nine patients were included in the study, which was performed retrospectively. The average age was 29 years. The mean defect size ranged from 1 to 3 cm². Most of the lesions were found on the medial side (n = 31), with a few on the lateral (n = 6) or tibial side (n = 2). After an average follow-up of 20 months, the Lysholm score was 92 points.

More recently, Imhoff and colleagues[29] presented their long-term results of 26 talar OATS procedures. The follow-up averaged 84 months. All patients completed the AOFAS, Tegner, and VAS scores. All scores improved significantly from preoperative to postoperative status. In addition, MRI was performed to judge the quality of surgery, but was found not to be useful in a standard setting to predict the overall outcome. The investigators concluded that patients who underwent an OATS procedure did benefit from the procedure even in the long term.

Why OATS is Favored

- Multiple studies have demonstrated better than 90% good to excellent results, with minimal complications and proven long-term results.
- An autograft eliminates the concern for infection and cartilage viability that is present with an allograft.
- OATS is a cost-effective technique and is available to all surgeons, unlike an allograft, which can be of limited availability.
- Despite the presence of occasional donor-site pain, the consistent improvement in function and pain of the ankle outweighs the risk.

ALLOGRAFT TALAR RECONSTRUCTION

Allograft reconstruction for OCLT was first reported by Gross and colleagues[37] in 2001. The 9 patients in this series had failed prior operative intervention, with 1 patient having undergone a prior OATS procedure for traumatic injury to the talus. Despite the need for fusion in 3 cases, 6 of the grafts demonstrated viability at a mean of 11 years from the surgery. Only 1 patient with an intact graft had pain, with the other patients pain free and able to ambulate for longer than 1 hour. Although this study did not demonstrate equivalent results when compared with OATS, the ability to use an allograft to reconstruct defects of any size or shape has sparked further interest.

Benefits of Allograft

- Ability to reconstruct a defect without limitations on width, depth, or shape. In patients with involvement of the shoulder of the talus, only an allograft can recreate the normal anatomy.
- Lack of donor-site morbidity. Iatrogenic knee pain in patients who have recurrence of ankle pain results in more dysfunction than was present before the index operation. Without a clear method of how to address the donor-site morbidity this is a concern, significantly so for larger lesions, whereby the rate of failure is higher and the donor-site morbidity is increased.
- Given that the entire talus is available, inadvertent damage to the graft or discrepancy in size of prepared graft to the defect is not devastating. The unaltered portion of the allograft can be used in these cases. Although the exact contour may not be available, it is a good alternative to closing the patient and performing the surgery at a later date.

Limitations of Allograft

- Diminished cartilage viability in comparison with an autograft is a significant concern. A fresh allograft stored in a serum-free modified culture medium revealed a decrease in viability of only 1.7% after 14 days in storage, but with a 28.5% decrease after 28 days.[38] Unfortunately, most tissue banks perform a 21-day screening process to minimize the risk of disease transmission. The grafts are not released until 3 days from completion of the screening, which makes the minimum time to implantation 24 days. However, additional time to schedule the procedure makes the practical delay very near or even beyond 28 days, which compromises the biological quality of the graft. Fortunately, the biomechanical properties of the graft do not deteriorate after 28 days from procurement.[38]
- Limited availability and cost limit the number of patients that can be treated. The cost of an allograft is not insignificant and occasionally is not covered by insurance, and therefore is not a viable option for every patient. In addition, given

the need to obtain a sized match graft, there can be a substantial delay for the patient, prolonging their period of disability.

- Disease transmission is a small risk; however, it can result in irreversible harm to patient. Although not reported in the literature for talar allograft, the risk of viral transmission cannot be assumed to be nonexistent, and the patient must be counseled on the theoretical risk.
- Immunologic reaction to the graft may adversely affect the viability of the transplanted chondrocytes. Giannini and colleagues[39] performed a biopsy of the transplanted cartilage in 7 consecutive patients who had undergone a bipolar allograft replacement of the ankle 1 year postoperatively, taken at the time of routine hardware removal. In each patient, the samples were histologically positive for catabolic factors such as matrix metalloproteinase (MMP)-1, MMP-13, and caspase-3. Although the clinical impact of this is not known, the presumption of the immunoprotected nature of cartilage may not be true, which may result in a more rapid deterioration of the transplant in comparison with an autograft. Corroborating this concern, in each sample taken the transplanted cartilage was more disorganized and had a lower proteoglycan content relative to normal articular cartilage.
- Inability to match the exact contour of the native talus. Although use of a size-matched talus can recreate the dimensions of the native bone, the radius of curvature in both the coronal and sagittal dimensions vary from patient to patient. This abnormal fit of the transplanted talus to the native tibia may result in increased shear stress and point loading of the graft, which may contribute to failure in the long term.

Indications and Contraindications

The indications are similar to those for OATS, but without the limitations based on size. Significant involvement of the shoulder of the talus is superiorly reconstructed with an allograft. Patients with a concern for underlying cartilaginous degeneration of the knee whereby obtaining a healthy autograft may be compromised, may be better served with an allograft. Patient with concomitant degeneration of the tibia are not candidates for isolated talar articular reconstruction. Use of a bipolar allograft has been described in such cases; however, this is not the focus of this article.

Surgical Technique

Smaller OCLTs that do not involve the bulk of the articular surface in the anteroposterior dimension should be approached as described previously for OATS. For large lesions involving a significant portion of the talus, a standard anterior approach provides excellent visualization and mitigates the need for an osteotomy. Given the ability to reconstruct the defect with a single piece of allograft, multiple options for preparation and placement are available. To match the contour of the native talus as close as possible to minimize abnormal forces to the graft, obtaining a preoperative CT scan is valuable. The CT scan allows for a more exact measurement of the native talus that facilitates the procurement company in obtaining a size-matched graft. Although using a graft that is not matched will minimize the delay to surgery, this is not recommended because this will lead to abnormal contact pressure with the native tibia and may lead to decreased long-term viability of the graft.

Graft preparation options

- Custom fit
  ○ The nonviable cartilage and bone is excised with an oscillating saw, minimizing excision of normal tissue. To adequately excise the OLT, perpendicular access

to the talar dome is required, which can be difficult if the lesion is more central. The defect is then measured and a matched allograft piece is fashioned. Typically this type of graft lacks intrinsic stability and must be fixated with 1 or 2 headless screws. This technique, though technically demanding, requires the least amount of excision of normal cartilage.

- Cylindrical plug
  - Following exposure of the defect, a guide wire is placed perpendicular to the articular surface at the center of the lesion. After completion of debridement, the maximal diameter of the lesion is measured. Using the provided instrumentation, the appropriate sized cylindrical reamer is chosen and the defect is cored out to a depth of at least 10 mm. The graft is then secured in the holder at a position that will allow for a similar angulation for placement of the guide wire. The matched donor harvester is used to create a matching donor graft. Following dilation of the recipient site to 0.5-mm dilation, the graft is gently impacted into place. No fixation is required in these cases, given the press fit that is achieved. The graft depth is carefully measured before placement to minimize the need for repetitive trialing of the graft, as this carries a risk of mechanical damage to the articular cartilage and can be difficult to do if the graft is too short and placed deep relative to the normal articular surface. This technique is less technically demanding than a freehand technique and does not damage the graft with placement of hardware; however, it will result in excision of a portion of the normal articular surface, particularly in cases where there is significant asymmetry between the length and width of the lesion. This approach is ideal for circular lesions on the medial or lateral aspects of the talus.
- Semicylindrical plug
  - A unique method to reconstruct large central and shoulder defects was described by Dragoni and colleagues[40] using the cylindrical reamers without the need for perpendicular access to the talus. The benefits of this method are the elimination of freehand graft preparation, press-fit technique, and the ability to reconstruct more central portions of the talus without the need to make a more aggressive osteotomy into the weight-bearing surface of the tibia. Exposure with a standard medial malleolar or lateral malleolar osteotomy is performed. Distraction of the joint with a pin-type distractor allows for excision of the defect, minimizing the risk of damage to the tibial articular surface. A guide pin is placed transversely through the shoulder of the talus parallel to the articular surface. The pin should be placed inferior enough such that greater than 50% of the circumference of the reamer is used. This maneuver creates a plug that has a larger bony diameter inferior to cartilage surface, allowing for press fit fixation (**Fig. 11**). The graft is harvested as described previously for a cylindrical plug, with dilation of the recipient site, and press fit into place. Minor adjustments are required to ensure an exact medial to lateral fit. This approach is ideal for a defect with a shoulder lesion, or for those that are larger in width than length and extend into the central portion of the talus. However, in such cases the shoulder of the talus will require violation if the large lesion is contained.

Anterior approach for large defects

- A standard anterior ankle approach is made between the anterior tibialis and extensor hallucis longus (EHL), or between the EHL and extensor digitorum longus, to avoid disruption of the anterior tibialis tendon sheath (**Fig. 12**).

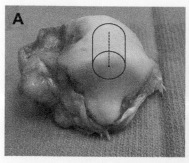
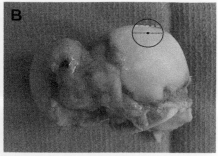

Fig. 11. Superimposed diagram of the technique for the semicircular plug as described by Dragoni and colleagues. The graft is taken from the lateral or medial aspect of the talus and directed centrally (*A*). By placing the center of the graft inferior to the articular surface, the center of the graft (*black dashed line*) is wider than the superior portion (*white dashed line*) (*B*). Although this creates less surface area for the cartilage, it allows for a press-fit technique.

- Placement of a temporary external fixator with a transfixation pin in the tibia and calcaneus facilitates exposure, in addition to minimizing the risk of inadvertent injury to the tibia during excision of the damaged talus (**Fig. 13**).
- Excision of the anterior 2 to 3 mm of the distal tibia, as would be performed with a cheilectomy, significantly increases visibility without creating instability of the ankle (**Fig. 14**).
- Based on preoperative imaging, the nonviable portion of the talus is excised.
  - A malleable retractor is placed superior to talus to protect the tibial articular surface. A small reciprocating saw is used to perform the osteotomy in the sagittal plane. A 0.045-inch (1.143 mm) K-wire can be placed from anterior to posterior and verified under fluoroscopy to facilitate an accurate cut.

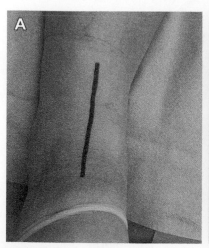
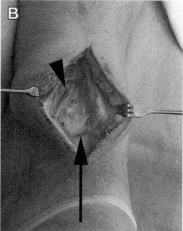

Fig. 12. (*A*) Incision for the anterior exposure for hemi-resection of the talus. (*B*) The neurovascular bundle (*arrowhead*) is deep to the EHL (retracted laterally). Following cauterization of the transverse vasculature (*arrow*), dissection is taken directly to bone and the neurovascular bundle taken laterally.

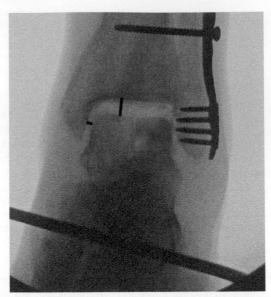

Fig. 13. Intraoperative fluoroscopy demonstrating the increasing the superior clear space after tensioning of the external fixator. The increased space facilitates placement of the saw and removal of the osteoarticular fragment while minimizing risk to the tibial articular surface.

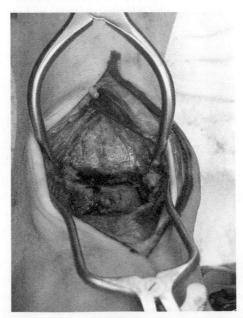

Fig. 14. Anterior tibial cheilectomy increases the exposure, facilitating placement of the reciprocating saw and removal of the diseased talus.

- ○ The malleable retractor is now placed in the gutter, and an oscillating saw is then used to perform the osteotomy in the transverse plane. To minimize inadvertent damage to normal talus, one can leave the reciprocating blade in place to act as a mechanical block.
- The talar fragment is then loosened to ensure that a complete cut has been made (**Fig. 15**). The fragment is then grasped with a towel clip or bone tenaculum, and removed en bloc (**Fig. 16**).
- The excised fragment is then measured for width and depth to prepare the allograft. In this case, given that the entire anteroposterior diameter will be replaced, the entire length is used (**Fig. 17**).
- The allograft is secured with the provided instrumentation and the measurement marked out (**Fig. 18**). Marking the graft with a 1-mm increase in both width and depth ensures that an excessively small graft is not created.
- Osteotomy is performed with an oscillating saw under cool irrigation to minimize heat necrosis. The authors prefer to make the initial cut from anterior to posterior in the transverse plane. Two 0.045-inch K-wires are then placed from dorsal to plantar, traversing this cut to prevent graft slippage after completion of the sagittal osteotomy. Although this damages the articular surface, loss of the allograft is a devastating complication and must be avoided at all costs. The osteotomy is then completed in the sagittal plane, followed by removal of the K-wires.
- The graft is trialed and adjustments made until the cartilaginous surfaces are flush. The graft can be secured back to the remaining allograft with 2 0.045-inch K-wires to provide a stable surface for making adjustments. The graft is very difficult to handle at this stage and must be secured before using the saw.

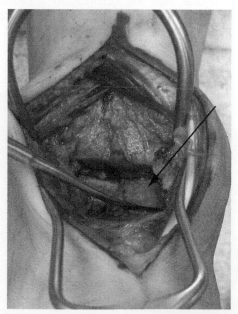

Fig. 15. A freer elevator is used to confirm that the osteotomized talus (*arrow*) is free of all bony attachment. If the talus is partially attached, removal may result in fragmentation, which increases the difficulty of resection and complicates obtaining an accurate measurement for the allograft.

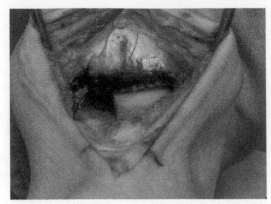

Fig. 16. Complete resection of the diseased portion of the talus has been performed. Visualization should confirm complete removal of the posterior segment of the talus.

- Following satisfactory sizing of the graft, the authors prefer fixation with 2 headless screws to minimize implant prominence and inadvertent damage to the tibial articular surface (**Fig. 19**).
- Addition of bone-graft substitute to the interface between the host bone and allograft has been described, and is performed by the authors to theoretically increase the rate of graft incorporation. However, no data exist to support its use for this procedure.
- Intraoperative confirmation of symmetric height of the native and transplanted cartilage is more critical than the radiographic appearance, secondary to a possible difference in the thickness of the cartilage (**Fig. 20**).
- Standard closure is performed, and the patient is placed into a well-padded splint in neutral.

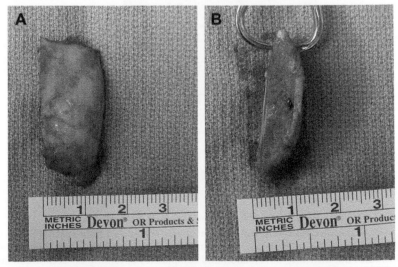

Fig. 17. The resected talus is measured for both width (*A*) and depth (*B*).

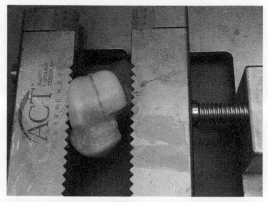

Fig. 18. The graft is secured in the provided instrumentation to provide a stable cutting surface and to eliminate the risk of graft slippage. A skin marker is used to mark the width and depth of the osteotomy required on the allograft.

Postoperative Protocol

- Patients are kept non–weight-bearing for 10 to 12 weeks postoperatively in a fracture boot. However, patients are encouraged to perform range-of-motion exercises and non–weight-bearing therapy that can be initiated at 2 weeks. Use of a fracture boot is continued on initiation of weight-bearing until bony trabeculation is noted between the graft and native talus. In a review of 15 patients who underwent large bulk allograft reconstruction, this was noted at a mean of 18.5 weeks.[41]
- Use of a lace-up ankle brace is recommended by the authors for up to 1 year following surgery to minimize the risk of trauma to the graft. Impact sports,

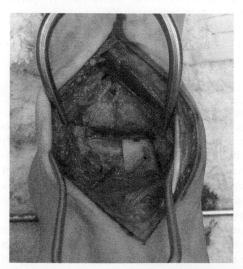

Fig. 19. Final appearance of the allograft in place. Two headless screws were used for fixation (circular defects within cartilage). Headed screws may be used; however, care must be taken to ensure that the head is placed deep into the cartilage surface to prevent damage to the tibia.

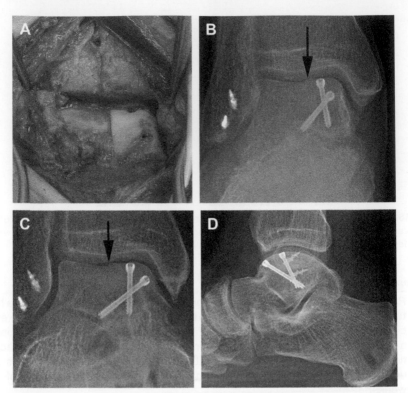

Fig. 20. Intraoperative appearance of the graft demonstrates that it has been placed flush to native cartilage (*A*). Radiographic appearance at 1 year demonstrates incorporation of the graft; however, note the elevated of appearance of the subchondral bone (*arrow*) on both the anteroposterior (*B*) and mortise (*C*) radiographs. The asymmetric appearance can be difficult to view on the lateral radiograph (*D*).

including running, is avoided for 1 year to minimize the risk of fragmentation and collapse.

Pitfalls

- Pitfalls similar to those described for an OATS procedure, with respect to the medial malleolar osteotomy and graft height, should be avoided.
- Damage or loss of the allograft can occur. In cases where the defect is less than 50% of the width of the talus, taking care to preserve the other half of the talus provides a secondary source of graft. Although it will not exactly match the contour, in such a complex situation it is the best alternative. Holding the graft secure with specially designed forceps or transfixing the graft to the remaining allograft will minimize the risk of loss.
- The radiographic appearance after graft placement may demonstrate a step-off of the subchondral bone. This appearance can be normal as long as intraoperative verification of a flush chondral surface has been noted. Discussion of this finding preoperatively and, if possible, demonstration photographically of the intraoperative appearance can avoid patient dissatisfaction during the postoperative period.

Results

Following the initial evaluation of allografting by Gross in 2001, Raikin reported his results of 15 cases of large defects with a minimum volume of 3 cm^3 and a mean volume of 6.059 cm^3.[41] Surgical approach was dictated by the size and location of lesion, with a medial malleolar osteotomy in 4 patients, fibular osteotomy in 1 patient, and an anterior approach with hemi-resection of the talar dome in 10 patients. All grafts were custom fit and secured with headless screws. Intraoperative articular congruity was considered to be more critical than achieving radiographic congruity secondary to variability in cartilage thickness. At a mean follow-up of 54 months, patients noted a mean improvement in the AOFAS score of 45 points. The greatest changes were noted in pain, activity, and walking distance. The mean improvement in the VAS score was 3.3 (range 1–8). Radiographs revealed resorption and/or graft collapse in 10 patients, without a clear correlation to the clinical outcome. Two patients required arthrodesis, one secondary to progressive arthritis and the other secondary to graft collapse. Eleven patients rated the results as good to excellent, and all patients would undergo the surgery again. All fresh allografts were implanted within 16 days of harvest; this relatively early implantation is, unfortunately, not possible nowadays given the stricter regulations. This study is the only one to date that has reported the results of any type of reconstruction for these very large lesions, and suggests a promising alternative to arthrodesis or replacement for this population.

Fresh allograft reconstruction for moderately sized defects (>1 cm and <2.5 cm in diameter) was evaluated in 13 patients by Hahn and colleagues,[42] with a mean follow-up of 48 months. Depth of the lesion was not used as an indication in this series. Ten patients had failed prior arthroscopic debridement, with the other 3 patients having lesions too large (2) or with avascular necrosis (1), and thus considered inappropriate for arthroscopic treatment. All grafts were implanted between 14 and 28 days of harvest. Following exposure (8 malleolar osteotomies performed), the native talus was debrided and the defect measured. A custom-shaped graft was used in each case and fixated with bioabsorbable pins, headless screws, or a combination of both. Emphasis was placed on intraoperative verification of cartilage alignment over the intraoperative appearance of the subchondral bone. The mean AOFAS score improved from 45 (range 23–65) preoperatively to 81 (range 61–95) at final evaluation. Eleven patients were able to return to high-impact sports, and all patients were satisfied and willing to undergo the surgery again. Although the series is limited by a small number of patients, the 100% graft-retention rate and patient satisfaction is encouraging.

The largest study reviewing 38 patients who underwent fresh allograft reconstruction in moderately sized lesions (mean 1.5 cm^2) was performed by El-Rashidy and colleagues.[43] Inclusion criteria included a failed prior intervention, surface area of greater than 2 cm^2 considered unsuitable for other surgical intervention, or a depth of greater than 5 mm. Surgical technique involved the use of a cylindrical graft with a press-fit technique. At a mean follow-up of 37.7 months, the mean improvement in the VAS and AOFAS was 4.9 and 26.5, respectively. The greatest changes were seen in the pain, activity, and walking components of the AOFAS score. Good to excellent results were noted in 73% of patients, with all but 2 patients willing to undergo the procedure again. Graft failure was noted in 4 of 48 patients, resulting in 2 prosthetic ankle replacements, 1 arthrodesis, and 1 bipolar allograft ankle replacement. Fifteen patients underwent postoperative MRI scans that demonstrated no signs of graft instability/graft incorporation in 10 cases. The overall rate of graft retention of 89.5% with good to excellent results of more than 70% is comparable to what has been demonstrated with autograft reconstruction.

SUMMARY

Both autograft and allograft reconstruction have documented success in the treatment of osteochondral defects of the talus. Universal availability and known chondrocyte viability makes autograft OATS an excellent option for recurrent, deep (>5 mm), or moderate-sized (<2 cm^2) defects. For defects with a large diameter, large cystic component, or heavily involving the shoulder of the talus, an allograft provides an excellent option. Familiarity with the risks of donor-site morbidity with an autograft and the problem with chondrocyte viability with an allograft are important factors to understand when making the surgical decision and when counseling the patient.

REFERENCES

1. Kappis M. Weitere beiträge zur traumatisch-mechanischen entstehung der "spontanen" knorpelablosungen (sogen. Osteochondritis dissecans). Deutsche Zeitschr Chir 1922;171:13–29.
2. Berndt AL, Harty M. Transchondral fractures (osteochondritis dissecans) of the talus. J Bone Joint Surg Am 1959;41:988–1020.
3. Scranton PE Jr, McDermott JE. Treatment of type V osteochondral lesions of the talus with ipsilateral knee osteochondral autografts. Foot Ankle Int 2001;22:380–4.
4. Raikin SM. Stage VI: massive osteochondral defects of the talus. Foot Ankle Clin 2004;9:737–44.
5. Becher C, Thermann H. Results of microfracture in the treatment of articular cartilage defects of the talus. Foot Ankle Int 2005;26(8):583–9.
6. Ferkel RD, Zanotti RM, Komenda GA, et al. Arthroscopic treatment of chronic osteochondral lesions of the talus: long-term results. Am J Sports Med 2008;36(9): 1750–62.
7. Hunt SA, Sherman O. Arthroscopic treatment of osteochondral lesions of the talus with correlation of outcome scoring systems. Arthroscopy 2003;19(4):360–7.
8. Schuman L, Struijs PA, van Dijk CN. Arthroscopic treatment for osteochondral defects of the talus. Results at follow-up at 2 to 11 years. J Bone Joint Surg Br 2002;84(3):364–8.
9. Chuckpaiwong B, Berkson EM, Theodore GH. Microfracture for osteochondral lesions of the ankle: outcome analysis and outcome predictors of 105 cases. Arthroscopy 2008;24(1):106–12.
10. Choi WJ, Park KK, Kim BS, et al. Osteochondral lesion of the talus: is there a critical defect size for poor outcome? Am J Sports Med 2009;37(10):1974–80.
11. Gobbi A, Francisco RA, Lubowitz JH, et al. Osteochondral lesions of the talus: randomized controlled trial comparing chondroplasty, microfracture, and osteochondral autograft transplantation. Arthroscopy 2006;22:1085–92.
12. Savva N, Jabur M, Davies M, et al. Osteochondral lesions of the talus: results of repeat arthroscopic debridement. Foot Ankle Int 2007;28(6):669–73.
13. Wagner H. Operative behandlung der osteochondrosis dissecans des kniegelenkes. Z Orthop 1964;98:333–55.
14. Schottle PB, Oettl GM, Agneskirchner JD, et al. Operative therapy of osteochondral lesions of the talus with autologous cartilage-bone transplantation. Orthopade 2001;30(1):53–8 [in German].
15. Peters PG, Parks BG, Schon LC. Anterior distal tibia plafondplasty for exposure of the talar dome. Foot Ankle Int 2012;33(3):231–5.
16. Flick AB, Gould N. Osteochondritis dissecans of the talus (transchondral fractures of the talus): review of the literature and new surgical approach for medial dome lesions. Foot Ankle 1985;5(4):165–85.

17. Sammarco GJ, Makwana NK. Treatment of talar osteochondral lesions using local osteochondral graft. Foot Ankle Int 2002;23(8):693–8.
18. Gautier E, Kolker D, Jakob RP. Treatment of cartilage defects of the talus by autologous osteochondral grafts. J Bone Joint Surg Br 2002;84:237–44.
19. Draper SD, Fallat LM. Autogenous bone grafting for the treatment of talar dome lesions. J Foot Ankle Surg 2000;39:15–23.
20. Tochigi Y, Amendola A, Muir D, et al. Technique tip: surgical approach for centro-lateral talar osteochondral lesions with an anterolateral osteotomy. Foot Ankle Int 2002;23(11):1038–9.
21. Martin TL, Wilson MG, Robledo J. Early results of autologous bone grafting for large talar osteochondritis dissecans lesions. Presented at the 29th Annual Meeting of the American Orthopedic Foot and Ankle Society. Anaheim, California, February 7, 1999.
22. Speck M, Schweinfurt M, Boerner T. Osteochondral autograft transplantation for traumatic and degenerative lesions of the talus. Presented at the 4th Symposium of the International Cartilage Repair Society. Toronto, Canada, June 15-18, 2002.
23. Borazjani BH, Chen AC, Bae WC, et al. Effect of impact on chondrocyte viability during insertion of human osteochondral allografts. J Bone Joint Surg Am 2006; 88(9):1934–43.
24. Huntley JS, Bush PG, McBirnie JM, et al. Chondrocyte death associated with human femoral osteochondral harvest as performed for mosaicplasty. J Bone Joint Surg Am 2005;87(2):351–60.
25. Patill S, Butcher W, D'Lima DD, et al. Effect of osteochondral graft insertion forces on chondrocyte viability. Am J Sports Med 2008;36(9):1726–32.
26. Hangody L. The mosaicplasty technique for osteochondral lesions of the talus. Foot Ankle Clin 2003;8(2):259–73.
27. Hangody L, Kish G, Modis L, et al. Mosaicplasty for the treatment of osteochon-dritis dissecans of the talus: two to seven year results in 36 patients. Foot Ankle Int 2001;22(7):552–8.
28. Hangody L, Fejerdy G, Toth F. Distal osteotomy of the metatarsal bones in the treatment of metatarsalgia. Magy Traumatol Orthop Helyreallito Seb 1991;34(2): 95–101 [in Hungarian].
29. Imhoff AB, Paul J, Ottinger B, et al. Osteochondral transplantation of the talus: long-term clinical and magnetic resonance imaging evaluation. Am J Sports Med 2011;39:1487–93.
30. Hangody L, Kish G, Karpati Z, et al. Treatment of osteochondritis dissecans of the talus: use of the mosaicplasty technique—a preliminary report. Foot Ankle Int 1997;18(10):628–34.
31. Valderrabano V, Leumann A, Rasch H, et al. Knee-to-ankle mosaicplasty for the treatment of osteochondral lesions of the ankle joint. Am J Sports Med 2009; 37(Suppl 1):105S–11S.
32. Paul J, Sagstetter A, Kriner M, et al. Donor-site morbidity after osteochondral autologous transplantation for lesions of the talus. J Bone Joint Surg Am 2009; 91(7):1683–8.
33. Reddy S, Pedowitz DI, Parekh SG, et al. The morbidity associated with osteo-chondral harvest from asymptomatic knees for the treatment of osteochondral lesions of the talus. Am J Sports Med 2007;35(1):80–5.
34. Hangody L, Feczko P, Bartha L, et al. Mosaicplasty for the treatment of articular defects of the knee and ankle. Clin Orthop Relat Res 2001;(391 Suppl):S328–36.
35. Baltzer AW, Arnold JP. Bone-cartilage transplantation from the ipsilateral knee for chondral lesions of the talus. Arthroscopy 2005;21(2):159–66.

36. Al-Shaikh RA, Chou LB, Mann JA, et al. Autologous osteochondral grafting for talar cartilage defects. Foot Ankle Int 2002;23(5):381–9.
37. Gross AE, Agnidis Z, Hutchison CR. Osteochondral defects of the talus treated with fresh osteochondral allograft transplantation. Foot Ankle Int 2001;22(5): 385–91.
38. Williams SK, Amiel D, Ball ST, et al. Prolonged storage effects on the articular cartilage of fresh human osteochondral allografts. J Bone Joint Surg Am 2003; 85(11):2111–20.
39. Giannini S, Buda R, Grigolo B, et al. Bipolar fresh osteochondral allograft of the ankle. Foot Ankle Int 2010;31(1):38–46.
40. Dragoni M, Bonasia DE, Amendola A. Osteochondral talar allograft for large osteochondral defects: technique tip. Foot Ankle Int 2011;32(9):910–6.
41. Raikin SM. Fresh osteochondral allografts for large volume cystic osteochondral defects of the talus. J Bone Joint Surg Am 2009;91(12):2818–26.
42. Hahn DB, Aanstoos ME, Wilkins RM. Osteochondral lesions of the talus treated with fresh talar allografts. Foot Ankle Int 2010;31(4):277–82.
43. El-Rashidy H, Villas D, Omar I, et al. Fresh osteochondral allograft for the treatment of cartilage defects of the talus: a retrospective review. J Bone Joint Surg Am 2011;93(17):1634–40.

Managing the Cystic Osteochondral Defect
Allograft or Autograft

Graham A. McCollum, FCS Orth(SA), MMED(UCT)*,
Mark S. Myerson, MD, Jacques Jonck, FCS Orth(SA)

KEYWORDS

- Osteochondral lesion talus • Osteochondral defect talus • Allograft talus
- Autograft talus • Massive cystic defects talus • Uncontained talar cyst

KEY POINTS

- Treatment of talar osteochondral lesions less than 150 mm^3 with microfracture and debridement techniques produces reliable and consistent results.
- Lesions greater than 300 mm^3 do not respond well to microfracture and are difficult to treat. Surgical principles entail replacement of the cartilage and bone defect with allograft or autograft.
- Large uncontained cysts are not amenable to autografting techniques because the anatomy is impossible to recreate, the size is too substantial, outweighing the donor site morbidity, and stability of the graft is not guaranteed. In these situations, osteochondral allograft is a viable alternative producing a near-normal talus.
- Occasionally, the disease process involves the subtalar or ankle joints, with secondary arthritis. In these situations, joint preservation is impossible and salvage with an arthrodesis and bulk osseous allograft is the only surgical option.

INTRODUCTION

An osteochondral lesion of the talus (OLT) is defined as a cartilage defect involving the underlying subchondral bone, usually situated on the articular surface of the talar dome.[1–3] Several different terms have been used to describe this condition, including osteochondral defect, osteochondral fracture, osteochondritis dissecans, transchondral fracture, flake fracture, and intra-articular fracture.[3] Kappis was the first to describe osteochondritis dissecans of the talus in 1922.[4]

OLT is a common occurrence after ankle trauma, with a 6% incidence of cortical avulsion fractures of the talus noted in a series of 133 ankle sprains and a 27.9% incidence

The Institute for Foot and Ankle Reconstruction, Mercy Medical Center, 301 St Paul Place, Baltimore, MD 21202, USA
* Corresponding author. Department of Orthopaedic Surgery, The University of Cape Town, Groote Schuur Hospital Observatory, Cape Town 7925, South Africa.
E-mail address: grahammac@discoverymail.co.za

of talar dome chondral lesions found in a series of 86 ankle fractures.[5,6] Bilateral ankle involvement is found in 10% of cases, with most of these lesions located medially. For this reason, a theory of osteonecrosis has been postulated, and a hereditary component might be implicated, because there is a high incidence in monozygotic twins.[7–9]

Berndt and Harty summarized the world literature regarding OLT in 1959 and formulated their well-known classification system (stages I–IV) based on standard ankle radiographs as well as experimental cadaver work, with trauma being the primary cause.[4] The use of scintigraphy, computed tomography (CT) scans and magnetic resonance imaging (MRI) has led to earlier diagnosis and better visualization of these lesions. Cysts of various shapes and sizes can occasionally be seen underlying these OLTs. Anderson and colleagues[10] recognized cyst formation in the subchondral bone of the talus as the progression of a Berndt and Harty stage I OLT by resorption of necrotic bone trabeculae. They used CT or MRI imaging to propose a new classification system, based on the Berndt and Harty classification system, by adding a stage IIA, which includes all lesions with cyst formation. Hepple and colleagues[11] reviewed 430 consecutive hindfoot MRI scans, which were performed over a 7-year period, and found 18 ankles with OLT. A retrospective review of the standard radiographs of these 18 ankles revealed that 5 had OLTs that were not visible on radiograph and therefore could not be classified using the Berndt and Harty classification. These investigators compiled a new classification system based entirely on MRI appearance, progressing in severity from stage I (cartilage damage only) to stage V (lesions with subchondral cyst formation). They noted that stage V lesions could present as the initial lesion, formed by subchondral crushing and secondary resorption of the necrotic bone, or it may be a distal end point on the scale of progression from a simple transchondral fracture with the formation of a cyst caused by deep, forceful penetration of synovial fluid into the subchondral bone. Nine of the 18 ankles in their series were classified as stage V (50%) and the investigators noted that these were the most symptomatic and most difficult to treat and had the worst outcome. Scranton and McDermott[12] postulated that the pathologic process of cyst formation underneath an OLT involves forceful extrusion of synovial fluid into the subchondral bone caused by repetitive impact from walking and a ball valve effect from the osteochondral defect. This blow-out osseous lesion fell outside the original Berndt and Harty classification both in terms of disease as well as treatment and was therefore grouped as stage V. Raikin[2] described a subset of cystic OLT, exceeding 3 cm^3 in volume. He noted that these lesions were not amenable to standard repair options because of the disproportionate large volume of talar dome involvement and significant loss of articular cartilage in some cases. He added a stage VI to the modification of the Berndt and Harty classification by Scranton and McDermott to incorporate these massive cystic lesions. This article focuses on the management of these massive OLTs, the Raikin stage VI.

PATHOPHYSIOLOGY OF CYST FORMATION

Despite increasing knowledge concerning cystic OLTs, the cause and pathogenesis are still not completely understood. Some lesions remain asymptomatic and inert, whereas others progress with persistent bone edema and large cyst formation. Better understanding of this process may enable intervention and arrest the process. Several theories regarding the pathogenesis of subchondral bone cysts have been postulated. One states that the extrusion of synovial fluid through a transchondral fracture into the subchondral bone causes the cyst to form. The ankle joint is extremely congruent and the articular cartilage on the talus is very thin compared with the knee, for instance. Thin cartilage is less elastic[13] and thus it has a high compression modulus and is less deformable. For this reason, it is not a good shock absorber and the subchondral bone of the talus is exposed to high-impact forces during loading and injury, predisposing to subchondral disruption. A disrupted subchondral bone plate is likely to be one of the major factors influencing the progression or arrest of cyst formation.[14] Articular cartilage is 75% water within a matrix of proteoglycans and collagen. It moves freely through cartilage, similar to a sponge, and compression disperses it to areas of less load. Because of the inelasticity and low deformability of talar cartilage, the pressure of the intracartilage water during loading is high, and a break in the subchondral bone plate forms a release valve for this pressure.[13] Cartilage water is a dialysate of synovial fluid and is interchangeable with the synovial fluid.[15] It continuously moves into and out of the matrix. High hydrostatic pressures within the subchondral bone cause osteolysis by interfering with local perfusion, causing local osteonecrosis.[16,17] This situation explains the development of cysts when the overlying cartilage is intact overlying a cyst. Cartilage not supported by subchondral bone loses proteoglycans and glycoprotein.[18] This situation enables water to flow more freely, with less resistance into the subchondral bone. Another theory postulates that a cartilage flap can act as a ball valve when there is a defect in the subchondral bone, allowing synovial fluid to be pressurized into the defect during weight bearing but restricting egress out of the bone, resulting in high intraosseous pressures.[12] Synovial fluid within the subchondral bone induces macrophage-mediated osteolysis and acidosis. However, not all subchondral cysts are associated with a transchondral fracture line and the contents of such cysts do not correspond with the histology of synovium.[19] Another theory postulates that a process of mucinous degeneration of intraosseous connective tissue, most likely triggered by trauma or local aseptic necrosis, causes the formation of subchondral cysts.[20] Raikin,[1] in his series of 6 massive OLT cases, had 2 cases of steroid-induced local osteonecrosis, showing a vascular cause for these large subchondral cysts.

Mechanical malalignment may contribute to progression of a cyst. Bruns and Rosenbach[21] showed the increased pressure load on the shoulders of the talus if the hindfoot or tibia was in varus or valgus. If there is a corresponding OLT, this is subject to significantly more point load and has been shown to negatively affect healing.[22,23] Spontaneous resolution of medial knee osteochondritis dissecans has been shown after high tibial osteotomy correcting mechanical varus.[24] OLTs after ankle fractures are common, and Thordarson and colleagues[25] showed the significant increase in talar contact pressure with malunion of the fibula. For these reasons, malalignment or malunion must be looked for and addressed if they are believed to contribute to increased focal talar load over an existing OLT. Ankle instability leads to repetitive trauma, increased focal load, and propagation of an OLT.[26] These conditions frequently coexist and must be examined for. Gregush and colleagues[27] showed that surgical treatment of ankle instability improved the healing of OLTs, but the clinical results and American Orthopaedic Foot and Ankle Society scores were inferior to ankle instability without an OLT.

A subset of these cystic lesions progress to become massive[1] (>3 cm^3) or become uncontained on the shoulders of the talus. The incidence of these massive lesions is not known, but OLTs are increasingly being recognized and are said to occur after 50% of all ankle sprains.[28] Considering that ankle sprains are common, occurring in 1/10,000 people per day and up to 5.36/10,000 athlete exposures, if only a small percentage progress to significant cystic lesions, they may be more common than previously appreciated.[26]

Massive lesions can be described morphologically as being contained and central, with adequate medial or lateral talar shoulders, or uncontained, with involvement of 1 of the talar shoulders. Some of these lesions expand distally and can involve the subtalar joint,[29] making surgical correction difficult, sometimes necessitating arthrodesis.

Clinically, most massive OLTs are symptomatic with deep ankle pain related to activity, intermittent swelling, and stiffness, with mechanical symptoms of locking, catching, or clicking. A fair range of motion is preserved, in contrast to osteoarthritis. Some patients remain asymptomatic despite significant disease. These patients pose a difficult treatment decision, particularly if the lesion threatens to involve the subtalar joint or destabilize the talar structure.

TREATMENT OPTIONS

OLT is often asymptomatic and, in general, is a slow progressive disease, which rarely leads to osteoarthritis of the ankle joint. Surgical treatment is usually indicated only in symptomatic lesions that fail conservative treatment.[30] Massive cystic OLTs are most often symptomatic and pose a treatment challenge for the foot and ankle surgeon.[11] Nonoperative treatment is usually indicated for ankles with no or minimal symptoms, Berndt and Harty stage I and II lesions, medial-sided stage III lesions, and lesions with intact cartilage on arthroscopy and includes rest, ice, limited weight bearing, and orthotics in cases with subjective ankle instability.[31] A review of the literature[31] revealed a poor rate of success of only 45%. Nonoperative treatment does not have healing potential in cases with massive cystic OLT and can serve only to alleviate symptoms. Nonoperative treatment options include activity modification, intra-articular steroid injection, and bracing with a custom-made molded ankle brace such as an Arizona brace. This treatment may be chosen for patients refusing surgery or who have a medical contraindication. Intra-articular injections with platelet-rich plasma (PRP) or hyaluronic acid (HA) can also be used as a temporizing treatment to alleviate symptoms for up to 6 months in ankles with stage I to III disease; however, its efficacy in large cystic OLT is uncertain.[32]

The size of these massive cystic OLTs reduces the structural strength of the talar dome, which can lead to collapse and increased point loading, with the development of kissing lesions on the tibial surface. No good data are available regarding the natural history and progression of massive OLT, but because the development of osteochondral lesions of the tibial plafond or cyst extension into the subtalar joint changes surgical options from joint-preserving procedures that aim to restore cartilage to the talar dome to joint-sacrificing surgery such as arthrodesis (ankle or tibiotalocalcaneal [TTC]) or total ankle arthroplasty, early surgical intervention is indicated for these lesions, even in the absence of significant symptoms.

Large OLTs are challenging cases to treat and rely on adequate imaging studies. Plain radiographs usually show a massive defect. Mortise and Canale views best show the talar dome.[33] Evidence of tibial plafond arthritis and involvement may be evident and could change surgical management. To accurately delineate the cyst morphology CT scanning is essential. Proximity to the subtalar joint, integrity of the shoulders, and structure of the talus are accurately shown. The distal tibial plafond is also visualized, showing evidence of early arthritis if present. MRI is less useful at showing the bony anatomy but helps to determine if there is overlying articular cartilage and what the condition of the cartilage is and if there is a kissing lesion or bone edema in the distal tibia.[34] For smaller lesions, for which bone marrow stimulating techniques, pinning of a loose fragment, retrograde drilling, or local cancellous bone grafting are contemplated, MRI can determine the size of the cartilage defect and the extent of bone edema.[35]

Treatment planning is determined by the patient's symptoms, the size of the lesion, the presence of adjacent joint involvement, and talar structure stability. With massive lesions, often the joint motion is preserved and if possible joint preservation should be attempted as opposed to arthrodesis or total ankle replacement. The surgical options are discussed and described later.

The principles of surgery are to revascularize the subchondral bone and stimulate the formation of fibrocartilage if a cartilage defect is present or to transplant autologous or allograft cartilage and bone.

Lesions less than 1.5 cm^3 are amenable to bone marrow stimulating techniques, and good results have been shown.[36,37] The long-term clinical outcome after this technique is inversely proportional to the size of the lesion.[38] Shoulder lesions have shown inferior clinical results to central lesions after arthroscopy and microfracture.[39] Once lesions gain a size greater than 1.5 cm^3, the clinical results are less predictable and alternative techniques should be used. Studies of osteonecrosis in the femoral head have shown that microfracture with multiple passes of a drill bit and debridement decompresses the subchondral bones, reducing intraosseous pressure.[40,41] This situation also occurs in the talus and is a possible explanation for the pain relief obtained. The subchondral bone is richly innervated by nocireceptors,[42] and the decrease in the intraosseous pressure and denervation of the bone may contribute to the decrease in pain after microfracture. The resulting fibrocartilage has inferior biomechanical properties compared with hyaline cartilage and it deteriorates over time. For this reason, large lesions (>1.5–2.0 cm^3) initially have good results as the pain generator is eliminated but then deteriorates as the fibrocartilage degenerates. Smaller areas of fibrocartilage have less load to bear and survive longer, with better clinical results.[43,44] Other negative predictors are advanced age, a history of repeated trauma, and the presence of osteophytes.[45]

Osteochondral transplantation enables the filling of larger voids, but at the expense of significant donor site morbidity.[46] Autologous chondrocyte transplantation is another option. The defect has to be contained with adequate medial and lateral talar shoulders for these techniques, otherwise the chondrocytes or the autograft are not stable. There is a limit to the size of graft obtainable from the knee, and the anatomy of talar shoulder lesions is difficult to reconstruct with multiple cylindrical grafts. Good surgical access to the talus is necessary for this procedure. The graft needs to be inserted perpendicularly, and thus tibial or fibular osteotomy is frequently necessary for this technique. Isolated cancellous bone graft is not an option in most of these cases, because the overlying articular cartilage is not present or degenerate and must be replaced. Structural osteochondral allograft is a reliable option for these massive cases. Gross and colleagues[47] first reported its use in 9 patients and showed good results and graft survival in 6 patients over 11 years. Three ankles had an arthrodesis for fragmentation of the graft. Since then, other studies with small numbers have shown encouraging short-term to medium-term results,[2,48–50] with improving pain and function scores, but with several failures reported too. In these uncommon situations, structural osteochondral allograft is the only option for joint preservation.

In certain situations, osteochondral allograft is contraindicated. When significant ankle or subtalar arthritis is already present, success of joint preservation is compromised. Arthrodesis or arthroplasty are the alternatives. Because of the often-significant bone loss from the cyst formation, these procedures can be challenging, requiring large structural bone grafting to achieve fusion or stable integration of a prosthesis.[2]

Several joint-preserving surgical procedures have been described for the treatment of cystic OLT.[51]

Pinning/Fixation

Loose articular cartilage with attached subchondral bone and a good vascular bed is amenable to fixation with pinning. Polyglycolic or polylactic absorbable pins are useful, not requiring removal. A recent study[52] achieved healing in 6 of 7 lesions with good clinical results.

Retrograde Drilling

In cases in which the articular cartilage surface remains intact with a subchondral defect, retrograde drilling is a revascularizing option. In addition to enhancing local blood flow and bleeding, the technique decompresses the cyst and should remove the contents.[53] Multiple passes of the drill bit using arthroscopy, targeting devises, fluoroscopy, and in some cases, computer-assisted surgery[54] causes bleeding and internal local recruitment of mesenchymal stem cells and growth factors. The sclerotic margins of the cyst are fractured by the drilling.[55] Retrograde bone grafting can be difficult because the graft is solid and has to be passed through a small drill hole. Insertion of calcium sulfate and iliac aspirate is easier because it is a fluid and encourages the cyst to fill in and heal.[56]

Bone Marrow Stimulation with or Without Bone Grafting (Microfracture, Abrasion Arthroplasty, or Drilling)

Bone marrow stimulation implies the creation of a bleeding bone surface in the base of an OLT by perforating the calcified layer of subchondral bone, or the nonbleeding base of a cyst, numerous times with an awl or a drill. In subchondral cysts in which the calcified layer is absent and the base is bleeding, abrasion arthroplasty with a power shaver or burr creates the same effect. The disruption of intraosseous blood vessels leads to the release of growth factors and the formation of a fibrin clot. Neovascularization of the lesion and the introduction of bone marrow cells follow and eventually lead to the formation of a fibrocartilaginous layer.[20] This is the surgical intervention of choice in cystic and noncystic primary OLT smaller than 1.5 cm^3.[51]

Stimulating the Development of Hyaline Cartilage (Osteochondral Autografts, Allografts, or Autologous Chondrocyte Implantation)

Larger cystic OLTs with involvement of the overlying cartilage need surgical intervention that fills the cystic defect with healthy bone and the cartilage defect with hyaline cartilage.

Osteochondral autograft transplantation involves taking 1 or more cylindrical grafts of healthy hyaline cartilage and underlying bone from the ipsilateral knee to fill a prepared osteochondral defect on the talar dome. The aim is to replace the damaged portion of talar dome with tissue that is similar to the original hyaline cartilage in mechanical, structural, and biochemical properties.[20] It is indicated for treatment of symptomatic OLTs larger than 1 cm diameter with or without underlying cysts or for secondary lesions that have failed primary surgical treatment.[57] This procedure can be performed either by an open approach or arthroscopically and can be performed using either a single, bigger osteochondral plug or multiple smaller cylindrical osteochondral grafts (mosaicplasty) to fill the defect on the talus.[3,20] When treating cystic lesions, the osteochondral grafts taken from the knee should be slightly longer than necessary to provide cancellous bone with which to fill the prepared cyst before insertion of the bone plugs.[51] The outcome of this procedure seems positive, with a good or excellent result obtained in 87% of cases according to a recent systematic review of the literature by Zengerink and colleagues.[51] However, no mention was made about the outcome of this procedure in cystic OLT specifically. Although the donor site defects in the knee fill up with cancellous bone and fibrocartilage, 12% of patients in this review presented with morbidity of the donor knee joint.[58] The most common symptoms are knee and patellofemoral instability during daily activities, as well as pain. The use of a single cylindrical osteochondral graft prevents the formation of fibrocartilage, as is seen in the open spaces between the multiple plugs used in mosaicplasty. However, the risk of donor site morbidity is higher when a single large cylindrical graft is harvested from the knee compared with multiple smaller grafts. The mosaicplasty technique, although technically demanding, also allows for a more accurate reconstruction of the natural curve of the recipient talar dome when compared with a single, larger osteochondral plug.[51] The use of this technique has not been well described in very large cystic OLTs such as the Raikin stage VI lesions, and the amount of graft that may need to be taken from the knee for these lesions precludes this as a viable treatment option.[1,2]

Autologous chondrocyte implantation (ACI) is a staged procedure that involves the arthroscopic harvesting of 200 to 300 mg of healthy cartilage, either from the affected ankle or from the ipsilateral knee as the first procedure. The harvested cartilage is transported to a laboratory, where it is minced and enzymatically digested and the chondrocytes are filtered out. The isolated chondrocytes are then cultivated in a culture medium to produce many biologically active chondrocytes. The second stage of the procedure is performed as an open procedure. In the case of cystic OLTs, the so-called sandwich procedure is performed. This procedure involves the preparation of the cyst with curettes and a high-speed burr, drilling the base of the cyst and then filling it with cancellous autograft taken from the iliac crest, tibia, or calcaneus to the level of the subchondral bone. The bone graft is then completely covered with a periosteal flap taken from the ipsilateral tibia. Another layer of periosteal graft is then secured to the surrounding cartilage and sealed with fibrin glue to create a watertight cavity between the 2 layers of periosteal graft. This cavity is filled with the highly concentrated chondrocyte graft. The high number of active chondrocytes between the 2 layers of periosteum creates a tissue layer with a high concentration of hyaline cartilage. The outcome of ACI seems generally favorable, with a successful result ranging from 72% to 90% according to the review by Zengerink and colleagues, but the results for the sandwich procedure for large cysts is not mentioned specifically. Certain factors make this procedure less attractive, including the financial burden to the patient/insurer, the need for 2 procedures (of which 1 is an open approach often using a malleolar osteotomy), the violation of a native joint if cartilage is taken from the ipsilateral knee, the technical difficulties in creating a watertight cavity in the restricted confines of the ankle joint, and ensuring that the fluid-based chondrocyte medium stays in the desired location to achieve its function. The use of a tissue matrix as a biological carrier medium for the cultivated chondrocytes obviates periosteal flaps and changes the chondrocyte graft from a liquid that is difficult to control to a more manageable malleable solid, therefore making this a more attractive option. Giannini and colleagues[59] described an all-arthroscopic technique for matrix-induced ACI (MACI) using a biodegradable scaffold made from the benzylic ester of HA (HYAFF-11 [Hyalograft C, Fidia Advanced Biopolymers, Abana Terme, Italy]) to hold the chondrocytes as they are inserted into the prepared OLT with the aid of a custom-made arthroscopic introducer. Defects that were more than 5 mm deep were first filled with cancellous autograft taken from the ipsilateral proximal tibia during the second stage of surgery. Of the 46 cases included in this prospective series, 25 had an excellent and 13 had a good outcome at 36 months' follow-up. Three follow-up arthroscopies revealed hyalinelike cartilage on histology that was in continuity with the surrounding native cartilage. A negative predictive correlation was found with increased patient age and previous surgical interventions. This is an interesting concept, but no data could be found on its use for large cystic OLTs. Biological scaffolds for MACI are not available for clinical use in the United States. ACI is in general not indicated for patients older than 55 years, because chondrocytes loses its biologic ability with older age.[3]

Osteochondral allograft transplantation is a good surgical treatment option for large cystic OLTs.[1,2,47,60] Osteochondral allograft transplantation is performed as an open procedure, with or without the aid of a malleolar osteotomy, in which the diseased portion of the talar dome is excised in bulk and a fresh talar allograft, preordered and matched to the dimensions of the recipient talus with the help of preoperative imaging (radiograph, CT, or MRI scan), is shaped to fill the prepared defect in the talus perfectly. It is often fixed with countersunk screws or bioabsorbable pins. This is the surgical treatment of choice for Raikin stage VI lesions. Some advantages of this procedure are the ability to accurately reconstruct uncontained lesions involving the medial or lateral shoulder of the talar dome, the absence of potential donor site morbidity despite the need for a high-volume graft, and an angle of insertion that does not have to be perpendicular to the joint surface. The 2 biggest concerns with the use of osteochondral allograft for treating periarticular lesions are the viability of the transplanted cartilage and the potential risk for a tissue rejection reaction.[61–64] Several studies have shown that freezing of a cartilage graft to extend its shelf life and decrease immunogenicity also decreases the viability of the chondrocytes. Osteochondral grafts should therefore be fresh (<14 days after harvesting) and preserved at a temperature of between 2°C and 4°C.[65–67] Donors should also be younger than 40 years to ensure limited cartilage wear.[66] Although HLA antibodies have been found in patients who have received osteochondral allografts, the clinical significance is still uncertain.[68,69] No HLA genotype matching was performed in any of the series of osteochondral allograft transplantation for cystic OLTs that were reviewed.[59,60] Strict screening for infectious agents according to the guidelines by the American Association of Tissue Banks ensures safety of the donor tissue.[70]

CASE DISCUSSIONS

Our experience with the surgical treatment of large cystic OLTs with significant cartilage involvement using fresh osteochondral allograft transplantation is discussed using 5 case studies.

The senior author evaluated all patients preoperatively. Important information was gained from the patient history, specifically age, symptom severity/restriction of daily activities, and previous treatment. Raikin excluded patients with open distal tibial growth plates and older than 60 years.[1] Physical evaluation focused on the ankle and hindfoot as well as the body mass index (BMI, calculated as weight in kilograms divided by the square of height in meters). Patients with a BMI of more than 35 kg/m^2 were also not considered for transplant.[1] All patients had a standard set of weight-bearing radiographs of the affected ankle performed, consisting of an anterior-posterior (AP), mortise, and lateral view as well as lateral flexion-extension views. The radiographs were performed with a marker of a known size on the ankle to calculate the magnification.[1] The position of the OLT on the lateral flexion-extension views, relative to the medial and lateral maleoli, influenced our decision to use a malleolar osteotomy as part of our surgical approach or not. All patients had a CT scan of the affected ankle preoperatively to accurately determine the size and position of the cystic lesion. MRI scans and bone scans were not performed routinely. Radiographic signs of generalized osteoarthritis of the ankle joint (joint space narrowing, periarticular osteophytes), tibial kissing lesions, and cyst extension into the subtalar joint were considered contraindications for osteochondral allograft transplantation. However, lipping of the anterior distal tibia and dorsal talar neck is not considered a contraindication to this treatment, but a cheilectomy of the anterior ankle must be performed during the allograft transplant procedure in these cases.

Case 1: Uncontained Posteromedial Shoulder Lesion

Preoperative planning

A 45-year-old patient presented with progressive right ankle pain and swelling. Standard weight-bearing radiographs of the right ankle revealed a large cystic lesion involving the central and posterior portion of the medial talar shoulder. Flexion-extension radiographic views clearly showed that the lesion was never fully uncovered by the medial malleolus through the arc of motion. A CT scan with coronal and sagittal reconstructions accurately showed the large cystic lesion, which involved the medial shoulder and medial wall. No extension into the subtalar joint was noted, and the remainder of the ankle joint seemed unaffected. This patient was found to be a perfect candidate for osteochondral allograft transplantation through a medial transmalleolar approach. The patient's radiographs and CT scan were sent to the local tissue bank and a fresh donor ankle with similar dimensions was found. The donor talus was never frozen but kept at 4°C in Ringer lactate solution. The surgery was performed as soon as possible after graft harvesting, because the viability of the donor cartilage starts to decline after 14 days.[2]

Surgical technique

The surgery was performed on an outpatient basis. The patient was positioned supine with no bump under the ipsilateral hip to allow easy external rotation of the leg intraoperatively. He received general anesthesia, and a popliteal nerve block was performed using a nerve stimulator. A single dose of intravenous broad-spectrum antibiotics was given at induction of anesthesia. The leg was exsanguinated by elevation, and a thigh tourniquet was inflated to 150 mm Hg higher than the patient's systolic blood pressure before skin incision. The skin incision was marked and centered over the medial malleolus, starting 5 cm proximal to the tip of the malleolus and extending distally for approximately 7 cm, with a slight anterior curve at the tip of the malleolus. Blunt subcutaneous dissection identified the saphenous vein and nerve, which were retracted anteriorly. The periosteum was incised longitudinally with a knife in the middle of the medial malleolus and elevated anteriorly and posteriorly to expose the entire medial malleolus and medial distal tibia. The position of the medial malleolus osteotomy was determined using a K-wire and fluoroscopy. The osteotomy was angled at 45° to the long axis of the tibia and extended from proximal medial toward the tibial plafond at the lateral margin of the talar lesion. Hohmann retractors were placed anterior and posterior to the distal tibia to protect the posterior tibial tendon and neurovascular bundle posteriorly and the soft tissue anteriorly during the osteotomy cut. The osteotomy was performed with a micro-oscillating saw onto the level of the subchondral bone, using the K-wire as a guide. Care was taken not to penetrate the cartilage of the tibial plafond with the saw, and sequential fluoroscopic images were used during the cut to accurately determine the depth of the saw blade. The last portion of the osteotomy was performed with a small osteotome and the medial malleolus was retracted medially and distally using a sharp bone hook. This maneuver gave excellent access to the talar lesion. The defect in the overlying cartilage was easily identified, and a small rongeur and curettes were used to deroof the cyst and remove the intracystic gelatinous material.

The cyst was carefully probed to accurately determine its margins. The entire cyst was then excised in a single block using the micro-oscillating saw. The excised portion involved the medial talar shoulder and wall. Bone wax was placed in the talar defect and carefully molded to represent the normal contour of the medial talar shoulder and wall. The wax mold was carefully removed and placed on the back table, where it served as a template for the osteochondral graft. The resected portion of the talar dome and the wax mold were measured, and a similar segment was marked out on the donor talus. The graft was removed from the donor talus using a micro-oscillating saw. Before insertion of the graft, the cut surfaces of the recipient talus were drilled multiple times with a 2-mm drill bit, and all remaining irregularities and small cysts were filled with cancellous bone graft taken from the donor talus. The graft was then positioned on the recipient talus to create a congruent joint surface with accurate reproduction of the medial talar shoulder. The graft was secured in place using 2 bioabsorbable pins, which were placed from medial to lateral, avoiding the weight-bearing surface of the graft. Congruence of the talar dome was confirmed under direct vision while the ankle was manipulated through full range of motion. Fluoroscopic images (AP, lateral, and mortise) also confirmed a well-seated congruent graft, which accurately recreated the medial talar shoulder. After thorough irrigation of the ankle joint with normal saline, the medial malleolus was reduced anatomically and fixed with 3 cannulated 4-mm titanium compression screws (Depuy, Warsaw, IN).

Postoperative radiographs and a CT scan of the graft and osteosynthesis of the medial malleolar osteotomy are shown in **Fig. 1**.

Case 2: Massive Central Lesion Involving the Subtalar Joint and Arthritis of the Ankle Joint

A 50-year-old patient presented with a long history of ankle symptoms after a sprain injury several years previously. The pain had begun to deteriorate over the past 6 months, with associated stiffness and swelling. Crepitus was noted on clinical examination, and there was a 20° ankle valgus deformity. Subtalar joint motion was reduced and painful. The CT scan taken reveals a massive central talar lesion, almost causing discontinuity of the bone. Together with the valgus ankle deformity, there was evidence of significant ankle osteoarthritis. The cyst penetrated the subtalar joint and the ankle joint. The body of the talus was almost entirely composed of cyst, with poor subchondral support (**Fig. 2**).

Joint preservation in this case is contraindicated because of the arthritic ankle joint and the subtalar joint involvement. For these reasons, a TTC arthrodesis with bulk allograft to fill the defect was chosen to realign the ankle and hindfoot and obtain a solid fusion.

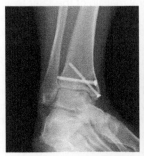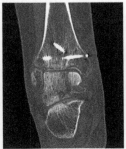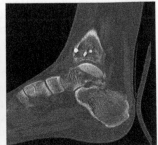

Fig. 1. Medial malleolar osteotomy and graft in place.

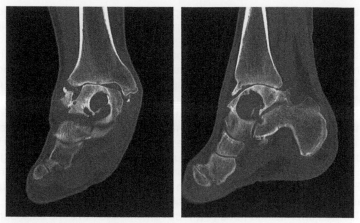

Fig. 2. Massive central lesion with osteoarthritic ankle.

Surgical technique

The ankle and subtalar joints were approached through separate incisions. To reach the large cyst and the tibiotalar joint, an anteromedial incision was performed exposing the medial two-thirds of the joint and talar body. The cyst was deroofed, and the remaining cartilage on the distal tibia and talar body removed with a flexible osteotome. The cyst cavity was curetted of fibrous and gelatinous tissue, and the perimeter perforated with a 2-mm drill bit to encourage intracyst hemorrhage. Care was taken not to cause a complete discontinuity of the talus body from head. The cyst was filled with a bulk allograft and compressed into the cavity flush with the remaining talus body. The posterior facet of the subtalar joint was approached through a lateral centered over the sinus tarsi. The posterior facet was prepared to good bleeding bone after careful distraction with a lamina spreader. A hindfoot fusion nail (Biomet, Warsaw, IN) was used for fixation. The nail was inserted retrograde through the calcaneus after guidewire placement and reaming. Good compression was obtained, with the locking screws and the graft well pressed into the cyst and the distal tibia (**Fig. 3**).

This patient went on to a successful fusion at 3 months.

Case 3: Large Anterocentral Cyst with Good Medial and Lateral Shoulders

A 40-year-old man presented with deep ankle pain related to mild to moderate activity. There was no recollection of trauma. The pain was associated with minimal stiffness

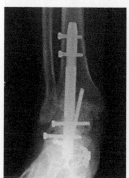
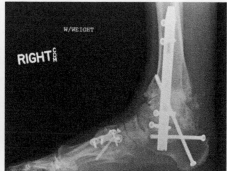

Fig. 3. TTC arthrodesis.

and swelling. There were no reports of crepitus, locking, or clicking of the joint. The pain was well controlled with analgesics as needed. He was referred after a significant OLT was identified on a CT scan.

The cyst was very large (>3 cm^2) and almost perforating the subtalar joint. Treatment decision making was difficult because of the mild symptoms and severe radiographic findings. The chance of spontaneous healing with conservative therapy was probably very low and progression expected. Intervening with a surgical procedure in this case was elected, because failure to do so with subsequent involvement of the subtalar joint or ankle joint would eliminate future joint salvage as an option. A bulk fresh osteochondral allograft was chosen, because the lesion extended to the subchondral bone of the subtalar joint and there would be no support for an osteochondral autograft from the knee and donor site morbidity would certainly be significant after such a large harvest. Preoperative flexion and extension radiographs showed that the bulk of the lesion was accessible anteriorly without a tibial osteotomy.

The ankle was approached through a 7-cm anterior incision. The extensor hallucis longus and tibialis anterior sheaths were preserved and the interval used to access the joint. The neurovascular bundle was retracted laterally. After an anterior arthrotomy and removal of the anterior lip of the distal tibia, the lesion was identified and probed. An oscillating saw was used to sharply excise the cyst down to the base, leaving both the healthy medial and lateral shoulders of the talus intact. The subtalar joint was not perforated. After cyst excision, there was a substantial central defect in the remaining talus (**Fig. 4**).

Accurately shaping a graft to fit in the defect is difficult without a mold or template. The edges are sharp, the floor is irregular, and the depth of the defect varies. To assist graft shaping, surgical wax was pressed into the defect to create a three-dimensional mold of the void and then carefully removed (**Fig. 5**).

The pliable wax is shaped by the contours of the defect. The mold is then used as a template to cut and shape the fresh allograft to fit perfectly. A small saw blade was used to perform the cutting of the allograft talus, ensuring accuracy. After insertion of the allograft, the cartilage should sit flush with the remaining cartilage. In this case, (**Fig. 6**), the graft was fixed internally with bioabsorbable pegs.

Fig. 7 shows a postoperative CT scan of the graft in situ, in a good position, with little evidence of subsidence and good early incorporation.

Case 4: Massive Uncontained Anteromedial Shoulder Lesion

A 58-year-old professional golfer presented with a 15-year history of ankle pain. The pain was activity-related and getting steadily worse, although at the time of examination, he was still able to get around the golf course without a cart. He denied a history

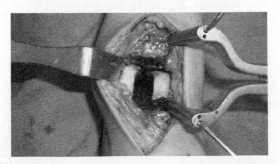

Fig. 4. Excision of the central cyst.

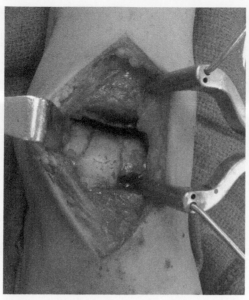

Fig. 5. Wax mold in place.

of trauma to the ankle. Radiographs revealed a large cyst in the anteromedial part of the talus, with an associated defect of the articular surface (**Fig. 8**).

The CT scan was even more impressive, showing the full extent of the cyst and the involvement of the talar surface as well as the very thin medial shoulder (**Fig. 9**).

The bone above the subtalar joint was also very thin, but the cyst had not perforated inferiorly. There were small anterior tibial osteophytes but the ankle joint was not

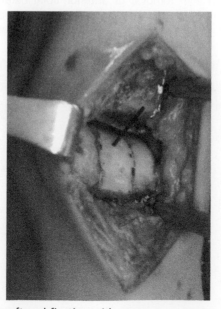

Fig. 6. Insertion of the graft and fixation with peg.

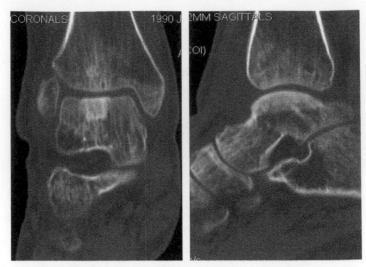

Fig. 7. Postoperative CT scan with central graft.

osteoarthritic. At this stage, there were no contraindications to salvaging the joint with surgery. Some might argue that this is aggressive surgery in the face of his minimal symptoms (he was able to walk a round of golf) but if left or treated nonoperatively, progression to subtalar and/ankle involvement would condemn this ankle and hindfoot to a fusion. Intervention before this stage is necessary.

This was a large, deep lesion with not much of a medial talar shoulder. Insertion of autologous osteochondral graft would likely have broken out the medial wall or would not have been contained in the talus. For these reasons, a fresh bulk osteochondral allograft was chosen. Although this lesion looked central and difficult to approach anteriorly, plantarflexion with removal of anterior tibial osteophytes exposed the defect adequately. Another advantage of using the bulk allograft is that the surgeon does not need exposure to get orthogonal with the talar surface, eliminating the

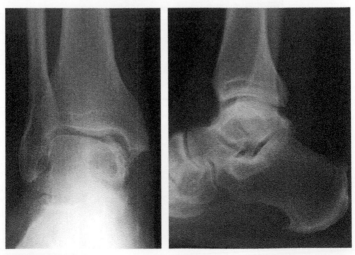

Fig. 8. Medial shoulder lesion.

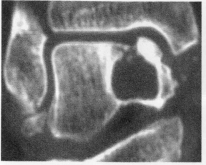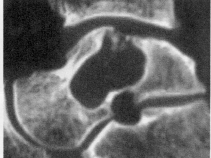

Fig. 9. CT scan of massive shoulder lesion.

need for a malleolar or tibial osteotomy in many cases. Osteochondral autograft requires insertion of the graft at 90° to the dome.

This lesion was approached through a 5-cm anteromedial incision, medial to tibialis anterior and avoiding damage to the saphenous vein and nerve. After osteophyte removal, deep plantarflexion and the use of a pin distracter, the lesion was identified and excised. The medial malleolar wall was paper-thin and was removed with the cyst, leaving a large defect. The defect was filled with a wax block and then carefully removed, creating a mold or template to fashion the talar graft to the perfect size and shape. The graft was secured with bioabsorbable pins.

Fig. 10 shows an anterolateral lesion approached through an anterolateral incision. After removal of the anterior tibial lip and osteophyte and insertion of a pin distracter, the joint is well exposed and the lesion addressed. In this case, if an osteochondral autograft was chosen a fibula osteotomy would have to be performed to get orthogonal to the lesion and the shoulder. An osteochondral allograft was used in this case.

Case 5: Large Posterolateral Lesion, Requiring Tibial Ostectomy

A 38-year-old patient had a painful ankle after an ankle sprain several years previously. The pain was associated with intermittent swelling and stiffness, which restricted recreational sporting activities. Radiographs and a CT scan showed a large contained lateral defect. Flexion-extension radiographs helped plan surgery by showing that the

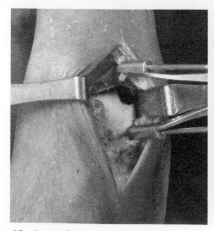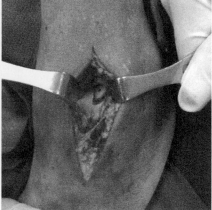

Fig. 10. Anterolateral shoulder lesion exposed.

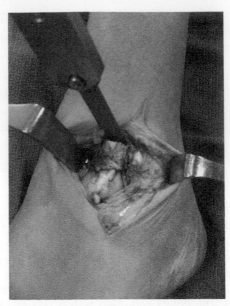

Fig. 11. Tibial ostectomy.

entire lesion was not accessible without an osteotomy. In this case, a lateral plafond window osteotomy or ostectomy was performed to access the entire lesion. It was impossible to reach the posterior part of the cyst without creating the window.

The ankle was approached through an anterolateral incision, taking care to preserve and retract the superficial peroneal nerve. The interval between extensor digitorum

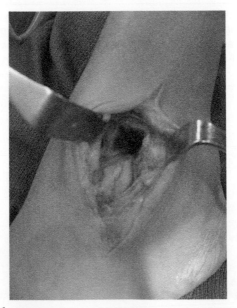

Fig. 12. Completion of ostectomy.

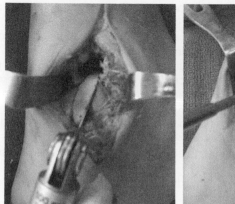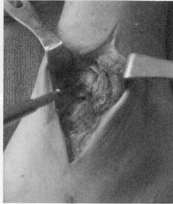

Fig. 13. Excision of the cyst and fixation of the distal tibial piece after grafting.

longus and peroneus tertius was used. An arthrotomy was performed, and the lateral part of the distal tibia and talus exposed. The defect was probed and the distal tibial cut marked to line up with the lesion and gain access. The osteotomy had 1 transverse and 2 longitudinal limbs to create a block of the distal lateral tibia. An oscillating saw was used to make the cuts down to the subchondral bone, and an osteotome completed the cut through the cartilage of the plafond. The transverse cut was angled slightly inferiorly, with the assistance of fluoroscopy to exit the distal tibia at the corresponding posterior part of the defect to gain exposure without going out the back of the tibia (**Fig. 11**).

The distal tibial piece can be removed, exposing the talus and the extent of the lesion (**Fig. 12**).

In this case, the lesion was excised and a wax mold of the lesion made using the technique described earlier, and an osteochondral allograft was shaped and placed in the defect flush with the lateral and medial shoulders. The free distal tibial piece was replaced after the graft insertion and fixed internally with a partially threaded titanium compression screw (Johnson and Johnson, Warsaw, IN) (**Fig. 13**).

SUMMARY

OLTs are generally benign and many heal or are not symptomatic. A subset of these defects progress to large cystic lesions, which have a less favorable prognosis. The treatment options are joint preservation or sacrifice, and the decision is based on the extent of talar collapse and involvement of the ankle and subtalar joints. Joint salvage entails either marrow stimulation techniques or hyaline cartilage replacement with allograft or autograft (from the knee or cell culture techniques). When lesions reach more than 3 cm^2 or Raikin class IV or become uncontained on the shoulders of the talus, autografting techniques become more challenging, with lower success rates and increasing donor site morbidity. Osteochondral allografting may be a better surgical option, often achievable without a malleolar osteotomy for exposure.

REFERENCES

1. Raikin SM. Fresh osteochondral allografts for large-volume cystic osteochondral defects of the talus. J Bone Joint Surg Am 2009;91(12):2818–26.

2. Raikin SM. Stage VI: massive osteochondral defects of the talus. Foot Ankle Clin 2004;9(4):737–44.
3. Zengerink M, Szerb I, Hangody L, et al. Current concepts: treatment of osteochondral ankle defects. Foot Ankle Clin 2006;11(2):331–59.
4. Kappis M. Weitere beiträge zur traumatisch-mechanischen entstenhung der "spontanen" knorpela biosungen. Dtsch Z Chir 1922;171:13–29 [in German].
5. Berndt AL, Harty M. Transchondral fractures (osteochondritis dissecans) of the talus. J Bone Joint Surg Am 2004;86(6):1336.
6. Aktas S, Kocaoglu B, Gereli A, et al. Incidence of chondral lesions of talar dome in ankle fracture types. Foot Ankle Int 2008;29(3):287–92.
7. Hermanson E, Ferkel RD. Bilateral osteochondral lesions of the talus. Foot Ankle Int 2009;30(8):723–7.
8. Woods K, Harris I. Osteochondritis dissecans of the talus in identical twins. J Bone Joint Surg Br 1995;77:331.
9. Erban WK, Kolberg K. Simultaneous mirror image osteochondrosis dissecans in identical twins. Rofo 1981;135:357.
10. Anderson IF, Crichton KJ, Grattan-Smith T, et al. Osteochondral fractures of the dome of the talus. J Bone Joint Surg Br 1989;71(8):1143–52.
11. Hepple S, Winson IG, Glew D. Osteochondral lesions of the talus: a revised classification. Foot Ankle Int 1999;20(12):789–93.
12. Scranton PE, McDermott JE. Treatment of type V osteochondral lesions of the talus with ipsilateral knee osteochondral autografts. Foot Ankle Int 2001;22(5):380–4.
13. Shepherd DE, Seedhom BB. Thickness of human articular cartilage in joints of the lower limb. Ann Rheum Dis 1999;58:27–34.
14. Qiu YS, Shahgaldi BF, Revell WJ, et al. Observations of subchondral plate advancement during osteochondral repair: a histomorphometric and mechanical study in the rabbit femoral condyle. Osteoarthritis Cartilage 2003;11:810–20.
15. Maroudas A, Schneiderman R. "Free" and "exchangeable" or "trapped" and "non-exchangeable" water in cartilage. J Orthop Res 1987;5:133–8.
16. Aspenberg P, Van der Vis H. Migration, particles, and fluid pressure. A discussion of causes of prosthetic loosening. Clin Orthop Relat Res 1998;352:75–80.
17. Astrand J, Skripitz R, Skoglund B, et al. A rat model for testing pharmacologic treatments of pressure-related bone loss. Clin Orthop Relat Res 2003;409:296–305.
18. Radin EL, Rose RM. Role of subchondral bone in the initiation and progression of cartilage damage. Clin Orthop Relat Res 1986;213:34–40.
19. Barth E, Hagen R. Juxta-articular bone cyst. Acta Orthop Scand 1982;53:215–7.
20. Han SH, Lee JW, Lee DY, et al. Radiographic changes and clinical results of osteochondral defects of the talus with and without subchondral cysts. Foot Ankle Int 2006;27:1109–14.
21. Bruns J, Rosenbach B. Pressure distribution at the ankle joint. Clin Biomech 1990;5:153–61.
22. Frenkel SR, Di Cesare PE. Degradation and repair of articular cartilage. Front Biosci 1999;4:671–85.
23. Flick AB, Gould N. Osteochondritis dissecans of the talus (transchondral fractures of the talus): review of the literature and new surgical approach for medial dome lesions. Foot Ankle 1985;5:165–85.
24. Koshino T, Wada S, Ara Y, et al. Regeneration of degenerated articular cartilage after high tibial valgus osteotomy for medial compartmental osteoarthritis of the knee. Knee 2003;10:229–36.

25. Thordarson DB, Motamed S, Hedman T, et al. The effect of fibular malreduction on contact pressures in an ankle fracture malunion model. J Bone Joint Surg Am 1997;79:1809–15.
26. Saxena A, Eakin C. Articular talar injuries in athletes: results of microfracture and autogenous bone graft. Am J Sports Med 2007;35(10):1680–7.
27. Gregush RV, Ferkel RD. Treatment of the unstable ankle with an osteochondral lesion: results and long-term follow-up. Am J Sports Med 2010;38(4):782–90.
28. Nelson AJ, Collins CL, Yard EE, et al. Ankle injuries among United States high school sports athletes, 2005-2006. J Athl Train 2007;42(3):381–7.
29. Van Dijk CN, Reilingh ML, Zengerink M, et al. Osteochondral defects of the talus. Why painful? Knee Surg Sports Traumatol Arthrosc 2010;18:570–80.
30. Myerson MS. Reconstructive foot and ankle surgery: management of complications. 2nd edition. Philadelphia: Elsevier; 2010.
31. Tol JL, Struijs PA, Bossuyt PM, et al. Treatment strategies in osteochondral defects of the talar dome: a systematic review. Foot Ankle Int 2000;21(2):119–26.
32. Mei-Dan O, Carmont MR, Laver L, et al. Platelet-rich plasma or hyaluronate in the management of osteochondral lesions of the talus. Am J Sports Med 2012;40(3):534–41.
33. Canale ST, Kelly FB Jr. Fractures of the neck of the talus: long-term evaluation of seventy-one cases. J Bone Joint Surg Am 1978;60(2):143–56.
34. Ferkel RD, Flannigan BD, Elkins BS. Magnetic resonance imaging of the foot and ankle: correlation of normal anatomy with pathologic conditions. Foot Ankle 1991;11(5):289–305.
35. Lusse S, Claassen H, Gehrke T, et al. Evaluation of water content by spatially resolved transverse relaxation times of human articular cartilage. Magn Reson Imaging 2000;18(4):423–30.
36. Gobbi A, Francisco RA, Lubowitz JH, et al. Osteochondral lesions of the talus: randomized controlled trial comparing chondroplasty, microfracture, and osteochondral autograft transplantation. Arthroscopy 2006;22(10):1085–92.
37. Becher C, Thermann H. Results of microfracture in the treatment of articular cartilage defects of the talus. Foot Ankle Int 2005;26(8):583–9.
38. Ferkel RD, Sgaglione NA. Arthroscopic treatment of osteochondral lesions of the talus: long term results. Orthop Trans 1994;17:1011.
39. Choi WJ, Choi GW, Kim JS, et al. Prognostic significance of the containment and location of osteochondral lesions of the talus: independent adverse outcomes associated with uncontained lesions of the talar shoulder. Am J Sports Med 2013;41(1):126–33.
40. Kiaer T, Pedersen NW, Kristensen KD, et al. Intraosseous pressure and oxygen tension in avascular necrosis and osteoarthritis of the hip. J Bone Joint Surg Br 1990;72:1023–30.
41. Specchiulli F, Capocasale N, Laforgia R, et al. The surgical treatment of idiopathic osteonecrosis of the femoral head. Ital J Orthop Traumatol 1987;13:345–51.
42. Mach DB, Rogers SD, Sabino MC, et al. Origins of skeletal pain: sensory and sympathetic innervation of the mouse femur. Neuroscience 2002;113:155–66.
43. Chuckpaiwong B, Berkson EM, Theodore GH. Microfracture for osteochondral lesions of the ankle: outcome analysis and outcome predictors of 105 cases. Arthroscopy 2008;24(1):106–12.
44. Cuttica DJ, Smith WB, Hyer CF, et al. Osteochondral lesions of the talus: predictors of clinical outcome. Foot Ankle Int 2011;32(11):1045–51.
45. Goldstone RA, Pisani AJ. Osteochondritis dissecans of the talus. N Y State J Med 1965;65(19):2487–94.

46. Lee CH, Chao KH, Huang GS, et al. Osteochondral autografts for osteochondritis dissecans of the talus. Foot Ankle Int 2003;24:815–22.
47. Gross AE, Agnidis Z, Hutchison CR. Osteochondral defects of the talus treated with fresh osteochondral allograft transplantation. Foot Ankle Int 2001;22(5): 385–91.
48. El-Rashidy H, Villacis D, Omar I, et al. Fresh osteochondral allograft for the treatment of cartilage defects of the talus: a retrospective review. J Bone Joint Surg Am 2011;93(17):1634–40.
49. Haene R, Qamirani E, Story RA, et al. Intermediate outcomes of fresh talar osteochondral allografts for treatment of large osteochondral lesions of the talus. J Bone Joint Surg Am 2012;94(12):1105–10.
50. Berlet GC, Hyer CF, Philbin TM, et al. Does fresh osteochondral allograft transplantation of talar osteochondral defects improve function? Clin Orthop Relat Res 2011;469(8):2356–66.
51. Zengerink M, Struijs PA, Tol JL, et al. Treatment of osteochondral lesions of the talus: a systematic review. Knee Surg Sports Traumatol Arthrosc 2010;18(2): 238–46.
52. Larsen MW, Pietrzak WS, DeLee JC. Fixation of osteochondritis dissecans lesions using poly(l-lactic acid)/poly(glycolic acid) copolymer bioabsorbable screws. Am J Sports Med 2005;33(1):68–76.
53. Taranow WS, Bisignani GA, Towers JD, et al. Retrograde drilling of osteochondral lesions of the medial talar dome. Foot Ankle Int 1999;20(8):474–80.
54. Citak M, Kendoff D, Kfuri M Jr, et al. Accuracy analysis of Iso-C3D versus fluoroscopy-based navigated retrograde drilling of osteochondral lesions: a pilot study. J Bone Joint Surg Br 2007;89(3):323–6.
55. Kono M, Takao M, Naito K, et al. Retrograde drilling for osteochondral lesions of the talar dome. Am J Sports Med 2006;34(9):1450–6.
56. Kennedy JG, Suero EM, O'Loughlin PF, et al. Clinical tips: retrograde drilling of talar osteochondral defects. Foot Ankle Int 2008;29:616–9.
57. Hangody L. The mosaicplasty technique for osteochondral lesions of the talus. Foot Ankle Clin 2003;8(2):259–73.
58. Reddy S, Pedowitz DI, Parekh SG, et al. The morbidity associated with osteochondral harvest from asymptomatic knees for the treatment of osteochondral lesions of the talus. Am J Sports Med 2007;35(1):80–5.
59. Giannini S, Buda R, Vannini F, et al. Arthroscopic autologous chondrocyte implantation in osteochondral lesions of the talus: surgical technique and results. Am J Sports Med 2008;36(5):873–80.
60. Dragoni M, Bonasia DE, Amendola A. Osteochondral talar allograft for large osteochondral defects: technique tip. Foot Ankle Int 2011;32(9):910–6.
61. Ohlendorf C, Tomford WW, Mankin HJ. Chondrocyte survival in cryopreserved osteochondral articular cartilage. J Orthop Res 1996;14:413–6.
62. Enneking WF, Campanacci DA. Retrieved human allografts: a clinicopathological study. J Bone Joint Surg Am 2001;83:971–86, 32.
63. Tomford WW, Duff GP, Mankin HJ. Experimental freeze-preservation of chondrocytes. Clin Orthop Relat Res 1985;197:11–4.
64. Marco F, Leon C, Lopez-Oliva F, et al. Intact articular cartilage cryopreservation. In vivo evaluation. Clin Orthop Relat Res 1992;283:11–20.
65. Tomford WW, Fredericks GR, Mankin HJ. Studies on cryopreservation of articular cartilage chondrocytes. J Bone Joint Surg Am 1984;66:253–9.
66. Malinin TI, Wagner JL, Pita JC, et al. Hypothermic storage and cryopreservation of cartilage. An experimental study. Clin Orthop Relat Res 1985;197:15–26.

67. Williams SK, Amiel D, Ball ST, et al. Prolonged storage effects on the articular cartilage of fresh human osteochondral allografts. J Bone Joint Surg Am 2003; 85:2111–20.
68. Meehan R, McFarlin S, Bugbee W, et al. Fresh ankle osteochondral allograft transplantation for tibiotalar joint arthritis. Foot Ankle Int 2005;26:793–802.
69. Phipatanakul WP, VandeVord PJ, Teitge RA, et al. Immune response in patients receiving fresh osteochondral allografts. Am J Orthop 2004;33:345–8.
70. Jacobs NJ. Establishing a surgical bone bank. In: Fawcett KJ, Barr AR, editors. Tissue banking. Arlington (VA): American Association of Blood Banks; 1987. p. 67–96.

Cell Cultured Chondrocyte Implantation and Scaffold Techniques for Osteochondral Talar Lesions

Ben Johnson, MBBS, BSc, Caroline Lever, MBBS, Sally Roberts, PhD,
James Richardson, PhD, Helen McCarthy, BSc, Paul Harrison, BSc,
Patrick Laing, MBBS, Nilesh Makwana, MBBS, FRCS(Orth)*

KEYWORDS

- Chondrocyte • Osteochondral talar • Lesions • Defects • Autograft

KEY POINTS

- Cell cultured techniques have gained interest and popularity in osteochondral defects because, unlike bone marrow stimulation methods, where fibrocartilage fills the defect, they allow for the regeneration of "hyaline-like cartilage" with better stiffness, resilience, and wear characteristics.
- Osteochondral defects (OCD) in the ankle are rare but are a challenging problem to treat in young active patients. If left alone, they can cause pain and reduced function and risk progressive degenerative changes in the joint.
- Most small OCDs of the talus, regardless of location, achieve good results with debridement and microfracture but lesions greater than 1.5 cm^2 have poorer outcomes when treated by these methods alone.
- The development of all arthroscopic techniques for repairing lesions, and the ability to cell culture from alternate stem cell lines, will alleviate the morbidity from osteotomy and, potentially, make matrix-induced autologous chondrocytes implantation a single-stage treatment.

Osteochondral defects (OCD) in the ankle are rare but are a challenging problem to treat in young active patients. If left alone, they can cause pain and reduced function and risk progressive degenerative changes in the joint. A variety of surgical procedures aiming to repair the cartilage defects have been used. Broadly speaking, these have involved simple arthroscopy and debridement, bone marrow stimulation techniques (microfracture, drilling, abrasionplasty), osteochondral transport (grafts, osteochondral autograft transfer system, or mosaicplasty), and more recently, cell cultured techniques (autologous chondrocyte implantation and matrix-induced autologous

Trauma and Orthopaedic Department, Robert Jones and Agnes Hunt Orthopaedic and District Hospital NHS Trust, Oswestry, Shropshire SY10 7AG, UK
* Corresponding author.
E-mail address: nilesh@bhanu.freeserve.co.uk

Foot Ankle Clin N Am 18 (2013) 135–150
http://dx.doi.org/10.1016/j.fcl.2012.12.008
1083-7515/13/$ – see front matter © 2013 Elsevier Inc. All rights reserved.

chondrocytes implantation). This article reviews the evidence on cell cultured techniques in talar lesions and presents the experience from the authors' unit (The Robert Jones and Agnes Hunt Hospital, Oswestry, UK) over the past decade.

Cell cultured implantation techniques were first introduced in humans in Sweden in 1987. Brittberg and colleagues described the first series of cases with lesions in the knee.[1] The technique involves harvesting cells from healthy articular cartilage and expanding the cell population in vitro before implanting the multiplied cells into the defect to allow for cartilage regeneration. Originally, the harvested cells were sealed into the defect under a periosteal graft. Collagen membranes are now also being used to retain the cultured cells. Matrix-induced autologous chondrocytes implantation (MACI) is a later development, whereby cultured cells are inoculated onto a 3-dimensional collagen scaffold in vitro, and this can be implanted into the defect.

Cell cultured techniques have gained interest and popularity in osteochondral defects because, unlike bone marrow stimulation methods, where fibrocartilage fills the defect, they allow for the regeneration of "hyaline-like cartilage" with better stiffness, resilience, and wear characteristics. It is hoped that this will help to improve long-term functional outcomes and prevent joint degeneration.

The authors' unit has the benefit of having an on-site laboratory with cell culturing facilities (adhering to cyclic guanosine monophosphate guidelines). This article reviews the current literature on these techniques and presents the author's experiences in the management of OCD using autologous chondrocyte implantation (ACI) and MACI.

PATIENT SELECTION/INDICATIONS FOR USE

Most small OCDs of the talus, regardless of location, achieve good results with debridement and microfracture, but lesions greater than 1.5 cm² have poorer outcomes when treated by these methods alone.[2] A systematic review of the literature in 2009 reported a mean 85% rate of success in the treatment with bone marrow stimulation in studies where the diameter of lesion did not exceed 1.5 cm.[3]

In accordance with evidence from the literature, the authors' approach is to carry out arthroscopic debridement and microfracture as a first-line treatment in lesions of all sizes and to consider progression to ACI/MACI as second-line treatment in cases that fail to respond.

Box 1 outlines the indications used for ACI at the authors' institution.

PREOPERATIVE EVALUATION

Assessment of the patient is aimed at identifying the size and location of the lesion and to identify any coexisting ligament instability or axial malalignment that may also need

---

Box 1
Indications for use of ACI in the treatment of OCD of the talus

Indications for autologous chondrocyte implantation of the talus

Any size symptomatic defect with failed previous surgery

Lesions greater than 1.5 cm² with/without cyst

Lesion with large cyst

Age between 15 and 55 years

No arthritis or bipolar kissing lesions

No instability, malalignment

to be addressed. Complete history and physical examination of each patient should be completed to ascertain the level of symptoms and degree of functional impairment. Standard radiographic examination, including antero-posterior and lateral weight-bearing views of the ankle, can demonstrate an irregularity on the talar surface, suggestive of OCD (**Fig. 1**) or large cysts underlying an OCD (**Fig. 2**) but the imaging modality of choice is magnetic resonance imaging (MRI) (**Fig. 3**).

Computed tomography (CT) can be used as an adjunct to delineate better the extent of the bone cysts underlying the OCD. In patients in whom previous surgery has been performed, such as microfracture or excision and debridement, the authors prefer MR or CT arthrogram (**Fig. 4**).

Single-photon emission computed tomography-CT (SPECT-CT) can be a useful investigation of patients who have undergone previous surgical intervention that has failed to relieve their symptoms. **Fig. 5** demonstrates a SPECT-CT performed in a patient after retrograde drilling of a bone cyst underlying an OCD. There is increased uptake within the OCD but more marked uptake within the sinus tarsi and along the line of the tract, suggesting this could be a source of the patient's pain after surgery (see **Fig. 5**).

ACI SURGICAL TECHNIQUE

ACI is a 2-stage procedure. The first stage involves isolation, culture, and proliferation of chondrocytes. Arthroscopy of the knee or ankle allows a specimen of cartilage to be removed and this is then used for chondrocyte culture. Although previously the authors' unit had taken specimens of articular cartilage from the trochlea or the superolateral femoral ridge, current practice is to harvest from the ankle. Harvesting from the ankle allows arthroscopic assessment of the ankle at the same time. Informed consent is acquired and viral testing is undertaken before biopsy procurement.

The first-stage arthroscopy involves standard anterolateral, and anteromedial portals are used. The lesion is evaluated; the status of the surrounding cartilage is assessed, and the cartilage defect is probed to determine the extent of any underlying

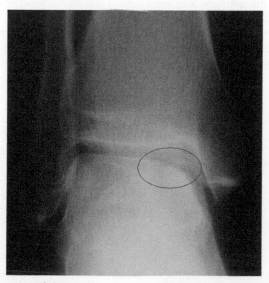

Fig. 1. Anterior posterior of the ankle suggestive of OCD on the medial aspect of the talus.

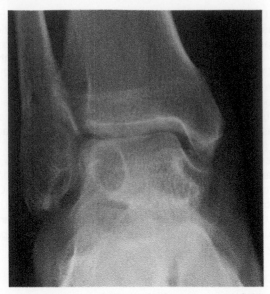

Fig. 2. Large bone cyst underlying an OCD on the lateral aspect of the talus.

bone defect. Sharp curettes are used to debride the lesion and remove pathologic tissue and unstable cartilage, which prevents damage to the surrounding normal cartilage. When bone cysts are shown on preoperative imaging, care is taken when probing the cartilage lesion to assess for any communications with the underlying cyst or scar tissue. If a talar cyst is present without communication to the cartilage lesion, then retrograde debridement of the talar cyst should be considered. This debridement can be performed at the second stage and bone-grafted retrograde (**Fig. 6**).

A 10 × 3 mm specimen of cartilage is harvested from the anterior margin of the talus, at the junction of the cartilage and neck, using a 5-mm curved notchplasty gauge. Approximately 200 to 300 mg is harvested (**Fig. 7**).

The sample is then transported to the on-site laboratory for chondrocyte culture. The port sites are closed using 4.0 nylon suture and a gauze, wool, and crepe dressing is applied. The patient is allowed to fully weight-bear following the procedure. Culture

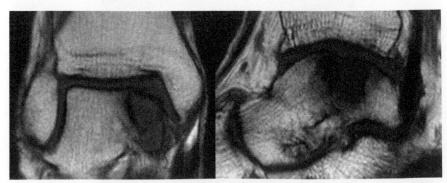

Fig. 3. T1-weighted coronal and sagittal images demonstrating the extent of the OCD seen on the radiograph in **Fig. 1**.

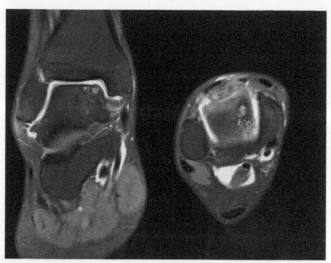

Fig. 4. Coronal and axial MR arthrogram showing OCD following previous treatment with microfracture.

of the chondrocytes takes 3 to 4 weeks. The techniques used for isolating and culturing chondrocyte have previously been reported.[4]

The second procedure is an open procedure and, depending on the location of the lesion, a chevron-shaped medial malleolar or an oblique fibular osteotomy is performed under fluoroscopic guidance to allow access to the medial or lateral aspect

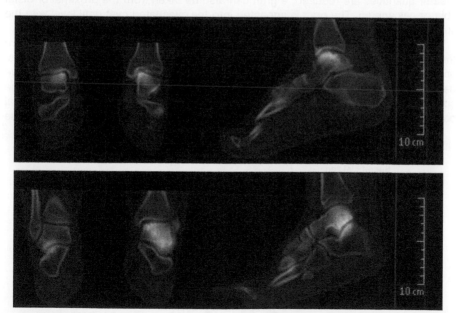

Fig. 5. SPECT-CT showing increased uptake on the medial talar dome of the talus in keeping with OCD and markedly greater increased uptake at the lateral aspect of the talus and along the tract of the retrograde drilling. Incidental increased uptake also seen in contralateral asymptomatic talus on the medial side.

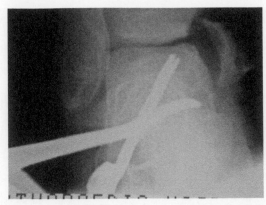

Fig. 6. Retrograde drilling of a medial OCD lesion with an intact subchondral plate. Retrograde bone grafting was also performed followed by ACI.

of the talus. The orientation of the osteotomy is important to allow adequate access.[5] The lesion is debrided to ensure a vertical rim of healthy articular cartilage using sharp dissection to prevent further damage to surrounding cartilage.

The subchondral bone is again inspected for any communication with the cyst. A hypodermic needle is useful for this. If a communication exists, then, using a curette, the subchondral cyst is debrided, removing any capsule or lining of the cyst (**Fig. 8**). The authors use bone graft for any defect that extends below the level of the subchondral bone.

Bone graft is usually harvested from the medial tibial plafond or lateral malleolus. If greater quantities are required, a graft can also be taken from the proximal or distal tibia or calcaneum. The graft is impacted into the evacuated cyst until level with the surrounding subchondral bone (**Fig. 9**).

Traditionally, cells have been implanted under a periosteal membrane taken from the distal tibia and secured with 6.0 vicryl sutures and fibrin glue. Within the authors' unit, this method was used for treatment of the earlier cases. However, studies have demonstrated that Chondrogide (Cell Matrix, Gothenburg, Sweden), a membrane consisting of porcine collagens type I and III is just as suitable for use as a periosteal patch during ACI.[6] Our current practice therefore is to measure the size of the base

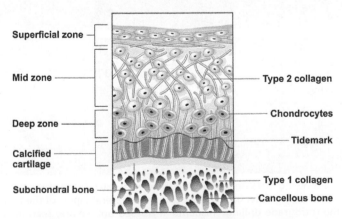

Fig. 7. The layers within a full-thickness cartilage graft taken from the talus.

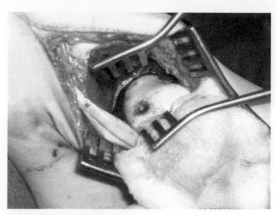

Fig. 8. Lateral talar lesion debrided to ensure a rim of healthy cartilage and the underlying bone cyst evacuated using a curette.

and superficial aspect of the lesion using a template and to cut 2 pieces of Chondrogide to size (**Fig. 10**).

The smaller piece is sewn over the bone graft surface with 6.0 vicryl interrupted sutures or fibrin glue is used to secure the edges. The second layer is then sutured with interrupted 6.0 vicryl sutures to the cartilage edges, leaving a small space for injection of the chondrocyte suspension (**Fig. 11**).

A pediatric canulae is used for delivery of the chondrocyte suspension, which is injected between the 2 layers of Chondrogide (**Fig. 12**). A final 6.0 vicryl interrupted suture is used to close the injection site followed by additional sealing with fibrin glue (Tisseel, Baxter, IL, USA) to create a watertight seal (**Fig. 13**). This procedure is also known as the "sandwich technique." If no bone defect is present, then the cell suspension is applied under the Chondrogide, which is secured within the defect using sutures and fibrin glue.

The osteotomy is reduced and the ankle is taken through a full range of motion. The ACI graft is reinspected to check for stability or delamination. If stable, the osteotomy is reduced and fixed. Medial malleolar osteotomies are fixed with two 4.0 Asnis cannulated screws (Stryker, Kalamazoo, MI, USA) through predrilled holes, and fibular

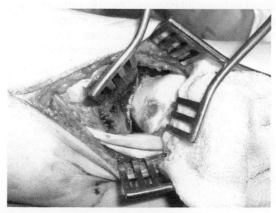

Fig. 9. Bone graft inserted to fill the cystic defect.

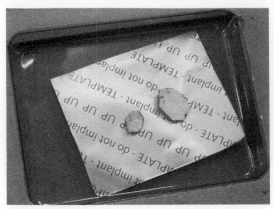

Fig. 10. 2 Pieces of Chondrogide (Cell Matrix, Gothenburg, Sweden) cut following templating of the base and the superficial aspect of the lesion.

osteotomies are stabilized with a lag screw and standard AO (algemeinshaft fur osteosynthesefragen) plates and screws. The wounds are irrigated and closed in a standard fashion. The patient is immobilized in a well-padded back slab.

MACI SURGICAL TECHNIQUE

The first stage of the MACI surgical technique procedure is the same as ACI with arthroscopic assessment of the lesion, probing of the defect, and harvesting technique. The harvested specimen of articular cartilage is placed in a sterile transport medium and sent in a cartilage biopsy transport kit to the cell culture laboratory (Verigen, Copenhagen, Denmark). Expansion of the chondrocytes in monolayer culture takes between 3 and 4 weeks. The cultured cartilage cells (15–20 million chondrocyte cells) are then inoculated onto porcine collagen type I/III membrane.

Access to the ankle to carry out the second stage is again by osteotomy of the medial malleolus or the lateral malleolus under fluoroscopic guidance. The lesion is debrided to ensure a rim of healthy articular cartilage, and a curette is used to expose and evacuate the subchondral cysts (**Fig. 14**). Bone graft is used to fill the defect left following debridement of the subchondral cyst. The lesion is then templated to guide the amount of the implant required to fill the defect (**Fig. 15**). The implant is fashioned to the size of the defect before implantation. The cultured cartilage implant must then be trimmed to match the defect size exactly and not protrude beyond the margins. More than 1 layer can be used if the defect is deep; the authors have used up to 2 layers. Defects that extend deep to the subchondral bone are bone-grafted and MACI placed on top.

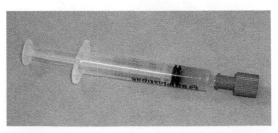

Fig. 11. Syringe that contains the cultured chondrocytes in suspension.

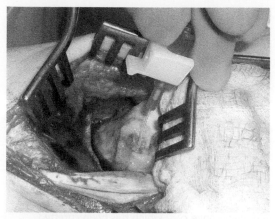

Fig. 12. Pediatric canulae used to deliver the cultured chondrocytes between the 2 layers of Chondrogide (Cell Matrix).

The implant is then fixed into the defect with 6.0 vicryl sutures and/or fibrin glue (Tisseel) (**Fig. 16**). The cell-seeded side is placed facing the subchondral bone.

If no bone defect exists, then the defect is filled using 1 or 2 layers of the MACI implant, which is secured in place using sutures or fibrin glue. The osteotomy is then reduced and fixed in the same way as for patients undergoing ACI, and the patient is immobilized in a well-padded back slab.

REHABILITATION

Following stage 1, patients are treated as they would be following standard ankle arthroscopy. Following stage 2, the early rehabilitation program is dependent on whether the patient has undergone osteotomy or not. All patients at the authors' institution have undergone an osteotomy to allow access to the OCD. Patients, therefore, are treated in a plaster for 2 to 6 weeks. At 2 weeks, if the osteotomy is stable, the patients are placed in an air-cast walker and an early range of movement is started with partial weight-bearing (PWB). Patients who have had treatment without an osteotomy can be fitted with an air-cast boot immediately and kept PWB for 4 weeks on crutches. Weight-bearing can be increased over the following 4 to 6 weeks until full weight-bearing is reached.

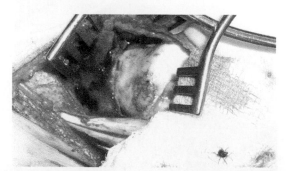

Fig. 13. Chondrogide (Cell Matrix) secured with 6.0 vicryl sutures and fibrin glue. The cultured chondrocytes lie between the 2 layers of Chondrogide (Cell Matrix).

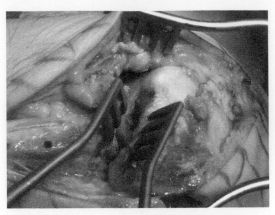

Fig. 14. OCD with underlying bone cyst, which has been curetted.

A phased approach to rehabilitation is adopted. By 6 weeks (phase 1), a pain-free full range of movement is aimed for. A heel toe gait PWB with elbow crutches is allowed. In phase 2 (6–12 weeks), exercises are given to build the intrinsic and extrinsic muscles of the foot. Patients are given isometric excercises to improve plantar and dorsiflexion strength. Weight-bearing is increased and hydrotherapy is commenced. The patient is able to return to sedentary work and can start driving a vehicle when pain-free.

During phase 3 (12–24 weeks), active strengthening of the ankle everter muscula-ture is developed as well as active ankle movements through all planes of movement. Full weight-bearing proprioceptive retraining is commenced and the degree of diffi-culty of the proprioceptive exercises performed is slowly increased. By 6 months, the patient is expected to have a normal gait pattern without pain and without walking aids. They should also have returned to work and nonimpact sporting activities. By 12 months postoperatively, patients would be expected to be able to perform all acts of daily living and walk up and down gradients and uneven surfaces without pain. Power walking, striding, and jogging are progressed and, gradually, recreational and sporting activities are introduced.

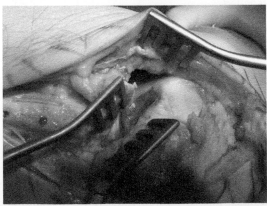

Fig. 15. Template taken of the cartilage defect to guide the amount of implant required.

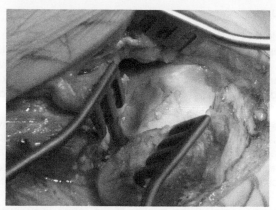

Fig. 16. The implant in situ following trimming. The implant is then secured using 6.0 vicryl sutures and/or fibrin glue.

CLINICAL RESULTS

Using the techniques described above, the authors have performed ACI in 34 cases and MACI in a further 18 patients. The clinical outcome was assessed using a combination of examination, patient satisfaction, and a modification of the ankle score of Mazur, Schwartz, and Simon. Patients were scored preoperatively and then yearly thereafter.

ACI

Thirty-four patients underwent ACI. Seventy-six percent were men with an average patient age of 38 (17–61). The right ankle was affected in 67.6% of cases and 68% of the lesions were medial. Previous surgeries included debridement alone, debridement and drilling, or microfracture, amd arthroscopic washout.

All patients had MRI ± CT before surgery. The average defect area was 185 mm^2 (66–400). Fifty-eight percent of patients had an associated underlying bone cyst. The average depth of the defect was 3.2 mm. The mean follow-up was 4.6 years (1–9). Assessment with a modified Mazur ankle score gave a mean preoperative score of 52 (16–70). The average postoperative score, at last follow-up, was 70 (29–90). The average satisfaction score was 3.4 (0 = "much worse" and 4 = "extremely pleased").

MACI

Eighteen patients underwent MACI. The right side was affected 77.8% of the time and the lesion was medial in 88.9% of cases. Average patient age was 35.6 (19–62) and 66.7% of the patients were men. Previous treatments included ankle arthroscopy alone, arthroscopy and bone graft of a talar cyst, microfracture, and arthroscopy and debridement.

The average defect area was 193 mm^2 (48–560). Sixty percent of the patients had an underlying bone cyst with an average depth of 3.6 mm. The mean follow-up was 6.8 years (4–8). Scores were available for 7 of the patients. Assessment with a modified Mazur ankle score gave a mean preoperative score of 38 (27–57). The average postoperative score at last follow-up for each patient was 70 (45–87). The average satisfaction score was 3.14 (2–4). All but 1 of the patients said they would have the procedure again knowing their status at final outcome.

HISTOLOGIC RESULTS

Biopsies were taken in 7 patients after ACI using a juvenile bone marrow biopsy needle, as close as possible to the center of the treated defect, to include the cartilage repair tissue and, where possible, the subchondral bone. Biopsies were snap-frozen in liquid nitrogen, embedded in OCT compound (Tissue-Tek, Zoeterwoude, Netherlands), and then cryosectioned to produce 7-μm-thick sections that were collected onto poly-L-lysine-coated slides.

Frozen sections were defrosted at room temperature and stained with either hematoxylin and eosin, for histologic assessment of the general morphology of the repair tissue, or toluidine blue, to indicate glycosaminoglycan content as per standard protocols.[7] Sections were then analyzed under polarized light microscopy to examine collagen fiber orientation and to distinguish between hyaline cartilage and fibrocartilage.

For 2 of the biopsy samples, the quality of the repair tissue was then analyzed histologically and scored using (1) the ICRS II visual analog scale (each of 14 parameters scored 0–10[8]), and (2) the OsScore (total score 0–10[9]), assessing the parameters listed in **Table 1**. A higher score in each scoring system represents tissue resembling healthy articular cartilage. These samples were taken 11 and 13 months following the second stage of the ACI procedure.

The overall score for each of the samples accessed with the ICRS II visual analog scale was 4.1 and 2.9 and the overall score following analysis with the OsScore was 8.1 and 6.9. Both repair tissue biopsies demonstrated a mixture of both hyaline cartilage and fibrocartilage, well integrated with the underlying bone. Neither biopsy demonstrated signs of inflammation, ectopic calcification, or vascularization, but chondrocyte clusters were observed in both.

The other 5 biopsy samples showed a mixture of hyaline and fibrocartilage in 2 of the biopsies and fibrocartilage alone in the 3 remaining samples. Fibrous tissue was not present in any samples. These histology specimens have yet to be formally scored.

Table 1
Scoring parameters used to analyze the quality of the repair tissue using the ICRS II visual analog scale and the OsScore

Scoring Parameter	ICRS II	OsScore
Tissue morphology	•	•
Matrix metachromasia	•	•
Cell morphology	•	
Cell clusters	•	•
Surface architecture	•	•
Basal integration	•	•
Calcification front/tidemark	•	
Subchondral bone abnormalities	•	
Inflammation	•	
Calcification	•	•
Vascularization	•	•
Surface/superficial assessment	•	
Mid/deep zone assessment	•	
Overall assessment	•	

COMPLICATIONS EARLY AND LATE

Typically low rates of complication are reported for both ACI and MACI. Of surgery-specific complications, the main issues are donor site morbidity (if harvested from knee), graft hypertrophy, graft failure, and associated morbidity from malleolar osteotomies, with occasional further surgery for the removal of metalwork.

ALTERNATIVE TECHNIQUES FOR CARTILAGE REPAIR?

Osteochondral transport techniques may also be used in OCD recalcitrant to debridement and microfracture. Where massive lesions exist, osteochondral allograft may be considered. Mosaicplasty where cylindrical osteochondral plugs are harvested from non-weight-bearing areas of healthy articular cartilage, usually from the knee and transferred into the defect, is another option in lesions greater than 1.5 cm, where bone marrow stimulation methods have failed. It has the advantage over ACI/MACI of being a single-stage procedure with a faster recovery and lower cost, but donor site pathologic abnormality can be more of a problem as a larger harvest area is needed. This larger harvest are limits the area that can be covered. An average donor site morbidity in the knee of 12% (0%–37%) across studies was noted in systematic review.[3] Another issue is that the resulting surface of the grafted area risks being uneven because of the different thickness of cartilage plugs with an irregular tidemark and "dead space" between the plugs that can fill with fibrocartilage rather than a hyaline type.

ACI

At present, studies into ACI in the management of talar lesions are, at best, level IV evidence of published case series. Differences in methodology and the use of a variety of outcome measures across the literature limit the conclusions that can be drawn. In addition, without having a comparison to other modalities of treatment in randomized trials, it is not possible to recommend cell cultured techniques over other methods of treatment at this point in time. However, the results from published case series show promising results with a tendency for clinical improvement.[10] Whittaker and colleagues reported results with ACI in 10 patients at 4-year follow-up. Eight of these patients failed prior arthroscopic treatment. At 4 years' follow-up, the satisfaction score was "pleased" or "extremely pleased" in 90% of patients. One of the larger case series on ACI of talar lesions presents 12 patients with 63 months of follow-up treating lesions of a mean size of 2.3 cm.[2] The American Orthopaedic Foot and Ankle Society improved from 43.5 preoperatively to 88.4 postoperatively, and all competitive sports players were able to return to full activity. There was no evidence on MRI of graft failure.[11–13] A meta-analysis, in 2011, reviewing 9 case series of ACI in ankle lesions for defects of a mean size of 2.3 cm^2 ($\pm$0.6), with follow-up at 32 months (range 6–120), showed an overall rate of clinical success of 89.9%.[14]

Despite small study samples, evidence suggests ACI is a valuable treatment option for focal cartilage lesions in the talar dome, especially in those patients in whom previous traditional surgical attempts of cartilage resurfacing have failed.

MACI

In respect to MACI, this is a relatively new procedure with results just emerging for short-term to midterm follow-up. Again, there are no comparative studies to other types of treatment; however, the current evidence does suggest improvement in patients' clinical symptoms following MACI treatment. There is no evidence as yet

Table 2
Summary of results of current studies of MACI in ankle lesions

	All Arthroscopic Technique	Number	Mean FU (mo)	Results
Aurich et al[18]	Y	19	24.5	50.3% improvement in clinical score
Magnan et al[19]	N	30	45	AOFAS improved 36.9 to 83.9
Giannini et al[15]	Y	46	36	AOFAS improved 57.2 to 89.5
Giza et al[20]	N	10	24	AOFAS improved 61.2 to 73.3
Schneider et al[21]	N	20	21.1	AOFAS improved 60 to 86.9
Dixon et al[22]	N	28	13	
Ronga et al[23]	Y	6	33.8	AOFAS improved 5 patients at 2 y
Makwana et al[24]	N	18	81.6	Mazur improved 38 to 70

that either technique has an effect on prevention of joint degeneration, and further long-term follow-up of the current cases is, therefore, required.

An all-arthroscopic procedure to perform MACI has been described whereby sutures are not needed and graft can be held in place with fibrin sealant alone. This procedure has the benefit of reducing morbidity from healing osteotomies.[15] **Table 2** summarizes the studies that have assessed patient outcome following MACI.

ADVANCES IN CELL CULTURE TECHNIQUES

Interest in alternative harvest sites is growing because this may reduce any morbidity from donor sites. Clinical studies have used chondrocytes from the detached articular cartilage fragment with good results in a series of patients.[15] However, no comparison studies to cells harvested from normal articular cartilage have been performed. Experimental studies have highlighted that chondrocytes from the detached fragment have inferior cartilage-forming capacity, opposed to those from normal articular surfaces.[16] Further investigations in this area are required to establish the full potential.

Future developments may also allow mesenchymal stem cells harvested from other tissues (eg, bone marrow) to be cultured and differentiated into a cartilage phenotype. The advantage is that the procedure is reduced to a single-stage surgery.[17]

Tissue engineering is also working toward improving the properties of regenerated cartilage. Chondrocytes from the different zones in the articular cartilage have been shown to have different mechanical properties and, therefore, emerging techniques to encourage growth of specific subpopulations of chondrocytes may further improve the clinical results of these techniques. Further research in this area is ongoing.

Several scaffolds can be used but they should be biocompatible and mechanically stable and able to support the loading of the cell source. Both natural sourced and synthetic scaffolds have been designed. Hyaluronan and collagen-based scaffolds are 2 of the most commonly used because these structures are naturally found in articular cartilage. Synthetic polyester scaffolds offer benefits in terms of reduced imunogenicity and better homogeneity and will likely be areas of further development in scaffold technology.

SUMMARY

The goal in treating osteochondral lesions is to develop a repair tissue that can withstand the mechanical loads of hyaline cartilage and integrate well at the interface with the remaining host tissue, with the aim that this will restore normal joint function and prevent future joint degeneration.

Clinical results of cell cultured and scaffold technology in the ankle, although still limited by small studies and midterm followup, are certainly encouraging. Results to date show improved functional scores following MACI treatment. The development of all arthroscopic techniques for repairing lesions, and the ability to cell culture from alternate stem cell lines, will alleviate the morbidity from osteotomy and, potentially, make MACI a single-stage treatment.

ACKNOWLEDGMENTS

The authors acknowledge the staff at Oscell and Andy Biggs in the medical illustration department.

REFERENCES

1. Brittberg M, Lindahl A, Nilsson A, et al. Treatment of deep cartilage defects in the knee with autologous chondrocytes transplantation. N Engl J Med 1994;331: 889–95.
2. Chuckpaiwong B, Berkson EM, Theodore GH. Microfracture for osteochondral lesions of the ankle: outcome analysis and outcome predictors of 105 cases. Arthroscopy 2008;24(1):106–12.
3. Zengerink M, Strujs P, Tol J, et al. Treatment of osteochondral lesions of the talus: a systematic review. Knee Surg Sports Traumatol Arthrosc 2010;18:238–46.
4. Harrison P, Ashton I, Johnson W, et al. The in vitro growth of human chondrocytes. Cell Tissue Bank 2000;1:255–60.
5. Nam EK, Ferkel RD, Applegate GR. Autologous chondrocyte implantation of the ankle: a 2 to 5 year follow UP. Am J Sports Med 2009;37:274–84.
6. McCarthy HS, Roberts S. Chondrogide® versus Periosteum: a histological analysis. Oral presentation, abstract No P007, British Orthopaedic Research Society meeting. Cambridge, June 27-29, 2011.
7. Roberts S, Menage J. Microscopic methods for the analysis of engineered tissues. In: Hollander AP, Hatton PV, editors. Methods in molecular biology, vol 238: biopolymer methods in tissue engineering. Totowa (NJ): Humana Press Inc.; 2004. p. 171–95.
8. Mainil-Varlet P, Van Damme B, Nesic D, et al. A new histology scoring system for the assessment of the quality of human cartilage repair: ICRS II. Am J Sports Med 2010;38:880–90.
9. Roberts S, McCall IW, Darby AJ, et al. Autologous chondrocyte implantation for cartilage repair: monitoring its success by magnetic resonance imaging and histology. Arthritis Res Ther 2003;5:R60–73.
10. Whittaker JP, Smith G, Makwana N, et al. Early results of autologous chondrocyte implantation in the talus. J Bone Joint Surg Br 2005;87(2):179–83.
11. Baums MH, Heidrich G, Schultz W, et al. Autologous chondrocytes transplantation for treating cartilage defects of the talus. J Bone Joint Surg Am 2006;88: 303–8.
12. Baums MH, Heidrich G, Schultz W, et al. The surgical technique of autologous chondrocyte transplantation of the talus with use of a periosteal graft. Surgical technique. J Bone Joint Surg Am 2007;89(Suppl 2, Pt 2):170–82.
13. Giannini S, Vannini F, Buda R. Osteoarticular grafts in the treatment of OCD of the talus: mosaicplasty versus autologous chondrocytes transplantation. Foot Ankle Clin 2002;7:621–33.

14. Niemeyer P, Salzmann G, Schmal H, et al. Autologous chondrocytes implantation for the treatment of chondral and osteochondral defects of the talus: a meta-analysis of available evidence. Knee Surg Sports Traumatol Arthrosc 2012; 20(9):1696–703.
15. Giannini S, Buda R, Vannini F, et al. Arthroscopic autologous chondrocytes implantation in osteochondral lesions of the talus: surgical technique and results. Am J Sports Med 2008;36(5):873–80.
16. Candrian C, Miot S, Wolf F, et al. Are ankle chondrocytes from damaged fragments a suitable cell source for cartilage repair? Osteoarthritis Cartilage 2010; 18:1067–76.
17. Gobbi A, Mahajan V, Karnatzikos G. Osteochondral lesions of the talus: current treatment dilemmas. American Academy of Orthopaedic Surgeons Annual Meeting Instructional Course Lecture Handout. San Diego, California, February 15-19, 2011.
18. Aurich M, Bedi HS, Smith PJ, et al. Arthroscopic treatment of osteochondral lesions of the ankle with matrix-associated chondrocyte implantation: early clinical and magnetic resonance imaging results. Am J Sports Med 2011;39(2): 311–9.
19. Magnan B, Samaila E, Bondi M, et al. Three-dimensional matrix-induced autologous chondrocytes implantation for talus osteochondral lesions. Presented at the 97th National Congress of the Italian Society of Orthopaedics and Traumatology. Rome, Italy. November 10-14, 2012.
20. Giza E, Sullivan M, Ocel D, et al. Matrix-induced autologous chondrocyte implantation of talus articular defects. Foot Ankle Int 2010;31(9):747–53.
21. Schneider TE, Karaikudi S. Matrix-Induced Autologous Chondrocyte Implantation (MACI) grafting for osteochondral lesions of the talus. Foot Ankle Int 2009;30(9): 810–4.
22. Dixon S, Harvey L, Baddour E, et al. Functional outcome of matrix-associated autologous chondrocyte implantation in the ankle. Foot Ankle Int 2011;32(4): 368–74.
23. Ronga M, Grassi FA, Montoli C, et al. Treatment of deep cartilage defects of the ankle with matrix-induced autologous chondrocyte implantation (MACI). Foot and Ankle Surgery 2005;11(1):29–33.
24. Whittaker JP, Smith G, Makwana N, et al. Early results of autologous chondrocyte implantation in the talus. J Bone Joint Surg Br 2005;87(2):179–83.

Autologous Matrix-induced Chondrogenesis in Osteochondral Lesions of the Talus

Martin Wiewiorski, MD[a,b], Alexej Barg, MD[a],
Victor Valderrabano, MD, PhD[a],*

KEYWORDS

- AMIC • Talus • Osteochondral lesion • SPECT-CT

KEY POINTS

- Recurrent ankle sprains and other trauma as well as ankle malalignment can lead to chronic osteochondral lesions (OCLs) of the talus.
- Several operative treatment techniques exist; however, the choice of the right procedure is difficult.
- This article presents a new surgical technique suitable for treatment of OCLs that combines bone plasty and a collagen matrix.

INTRODUCTION

Recurrent ankle sprains are frequently encountered in young people active in sports. Although acute ankle sprains are known to cause acute talar chondral lesions,[1] chronic instability resulting from recurrent sprains is suspected as the major cause of chronic talar osteochondral lesions (OCLs).[2]

Previous trauma is reported as the main cause of OCLs in lateral lesions (93%–98%) and less so in medial lesions (61%–70%).[3,4] Nontraumatic OCLs have been described in identical twins and siblings.[5,6] Etiologic factors other than genetics include talar malrotation/tilt (medial-posterior talar OCLs in posterior tibial tendon insufficiency or medial ankle instability), ankle malalignment (posttraumatic varus or valgus ankle), ischemia with necrosis, and endocrine or vascular factors.[3,7,8]

Conservative treatment fails frequently.[8–10] Common operative treatment methods include débridement and microfracturing,[11] osteochondral autograft transfer system

Disclosure: The authors have nothing to disclose.
[a] Orthopaedic Department, University Hospital of Basel, Spitalstrasse 21, Basel 4031, Switzerland; [b] Center for Advanced Orthopedic Studies, Beth Israel Deaconess Medical Center, Harvard Medical School, 330 Brookline Avenue, Boston, MA 02215, USA
* Corresponding author. Orthopaedic Department, University Hospital of Basel, Spitalstrasse 21, Basel 4031, Switzerland.
E-mail address: vvalderrabano@uhbs.ch

Foot Ankle Clin N Am 18 (2013) 151–158
http://dx.doi.org/10.1016/j.fcl.2012.12.009
1083-7515/13/$ – see front matter © 2013 Elsevier Inc. All rights reserved.

and mosaicplasty,[12–14] matrix-induced autologous chondrocyte transplantation,[15] autologous chondrocyte implantation,[16] and bulk allograft transplantation.[17] Although good results have been reported, only two of those techniques (osteochondral autograft transfer system and allograft) take into account the reconstruction of large bony defect present in large cystic lesions.

The aim of this article is to demonstrate a novel treatment approach for OCLs of the talus following the principle of the autologous matrix-induced chondrogenesis (AMIC). This technique was first reported by Behrens and colleagues[18,19] in 2005 and 2006 for treatment of full-thickness chondral lesions in the knee joints. An acellular collagen I/III matrix is placed onto the blood clot generated by microfracturing to provide a suitable environment for cartilage regeneration. Clinical results with up to 5 years' follow-up were encouraging.[20] Contrary to knee cartilage lesions, OCL of the talus often involves degeneration of the subchondral bone tissue. Large cysts are frequently found and need to be addressed during surgery. The authors, therefore, modified the existing AMIC technique by adding an additional step to reconstruct the bony defect after débridement of the cysts. Spongiosa is harvested from a suitable site (iliac crest or distal tibia [through the medial malleolus osteotomy window]) and is used to fill out the defect. The collagen matrix is placed on top to seal the spongiosa from the joint cavity.

Indications and Contraindications

Inclusion criteria
- Purely chondral and OCLs
- All stages according to the CT classification by Hepple and colleagues[21]
- Lesion >1.0 cm^2
- Patients ages 18 to 55 years
- Primary and revision procedure

Exclusion criteria
- Metabolic arthropathies
- Kissing lesions
- Major, nonreconstructable defects
- Noncorrectable hindfoot malalignment
- Chronic inflammatory systemic disorders
- Obesity (body mass index >30)

Preoperative Planning

Clinical examination of the ankle joint includes documentation of range of motion, sagittal and inversion/eversion stability, location of pressure pain, and alignment of the hindfoot.

Initial diagnostic imaging of the foot and ankle consist of plain radiographs (weight-bearing standard anteroposterior/lateral radiographs, Saltzman and el-Khoury view[22]) to assess alignment and exclude other pathologies than an OCL. MRI is performed to examine the condition of the cartilage and accompanying soft tissue pathologies. To adequately assess the extent of the bony lesion and amount of remodeling activity, the authors additionally perform a technetium Tc 99m dicarboxypropane diphosphonate single-photon emission CT–CT (SPECT-CT). Integrated hybrid systems like the SPECT-CT are a new approach, allowing acquisition of functional SPECT and anatomic CT images in a single diagnostic procedure.[23] The authors use SPECT-CT as part of a routine algorithm for diagnostics of all degenerative joint disease of the foot and ankle joints.[24] In cases of no scintigraphic uptake at the OCL, the lesion is not surgically addressed and the focus of surgical treatment is on instability and malalignment correction.

Operative Technique

The procedure can be performed either in spinal or general anesthesia in supine position. A tourniquet is applied. An initial arthroscopy of the ankle joint is performed to verify the size and location of the defect and the condition of the lateral and medial ankle ligaments. A standard anteromedial or anterolateral approach for arthrotomy is used, depending on OCL location (**Fig. 1**A). If the OCL cannot be accessed after capsular incision, a malleolar osteotomy should be performed. After the lesion has been exposed, the defective cartilage and the typically necrotic and sclerotic bony lesion underneath need to be débrided and microdrilled (see **Fig. 1**B–D). In cases of subchondral cysts, the fibrotic tissue within the cysts needs to be fully removed and the sclerotic cyst walls microdrilled. Sequentially, spongiosa bone is harvested from the iliac crest (alternatively, the distal tibia through the medial malleolus osteotomy) (see **Fig. 1**E). The spongiosa is impacted into the bony defect to fill it up. Next, a commercially available acellular collagen I/III matrix of porcine origin (Chondro-Gide, Geistlich Surgery, Wolhusen, Switzerland) is prepared. An aluminum template is used to determine the size of the lesion on the talus situs. The matrix is cut to size and then glued over the spongiosa with commercially available fibrin glue (Tissucol, Baxter, Deerfield, Illinois). For the knee joint, Drobnic and colleagues[25] showed that fibrin glue fixation provides primary stability, which is comparable to suture fixation of a collagen membrane. Care is taken not to overlap the surrounding healthy cartilage with the matrix (see **Fig. 1**F). Then, the ankle is moved several times throughout the whole range of motion and correct positioning of the membrane is checked.

If preoperative examination and radiographs show malalignment of the hindfoot, corrective osteotomies (calcaneal or supramalleolar) can be performed.[26,27] If ankle joint instability is noted during clinical examination and confirmed by ankle arthroscopy, ligament repair using a modified Brostrom-Gould procedure is recommended.[28]

Postoperative Care

Postoperative care consists of immobilization using a walker (Aircast Walker, DJO Global, Vista, California) and functional physiotherapy with 15 kg partial weight bearing, maximal range of motion of 20° with a continuous passive motion machine, and lymphatic drainage massage for the first 6 weeks. This initial phase is followed by an intensive rehabilitation phase with progression to full weight bearing and strengthening of the ankle joint stabilizing lower leg muscles and proprioception training for the following 6 weeks (up to 12 weeks). The patients are seen in anthe outpatient clinic 6 and 12 weeks after the surgery for a clinical follow-up examination and conventional radiographs. After 12 weeks, light sports exercising (swimming and cycling) are allowed. Return to competitive sports after 5 to 6 months. Postoperative care is identical for cases with corrective osteotomy and/or ligament reconstruction.

DISCUSSION

Only a few reports exist evaluating the clinical outcome after AMIC-aided treatment of talar OCL. The technique was initially described in a case report by Wiewiorski and colleagues in 2011.[29] Valderrabano and colleagues[30] reported approximately 15 cases

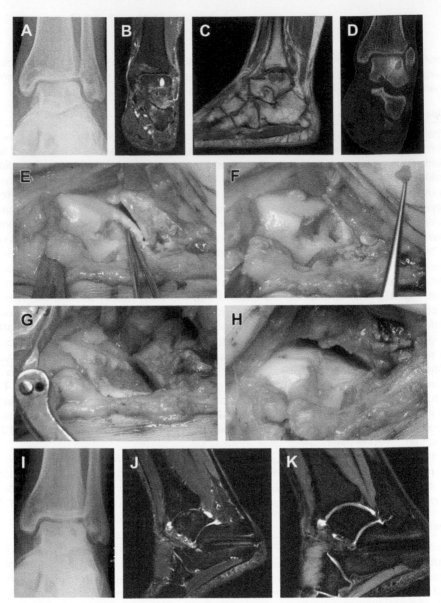

Fig. 1. Case of a 25-year-old man with posttraumatic OCL. Preoperative imaging (*A–D*): conventional radiographs (*A*) show a large partly detached fragment at the lateral talar edge; MRI with frontal fat-supressed T1 images (*B*) reveals the cystic nature of the lesion, whereas sagittal T2 images (*C*) show the centrolateral location and impressing anteroposterior extent and depth of the lesion; and SPECT-CT shows highly increased bone uptake in and around the lesion (*D*). The total volume of the bony defect was calculated as 7054 mm³. Surgical procedure (*E–H*): arthotomy revealed a highly unstable osteochondral fragment, which was bluntly removed (*E*); the subchondral cysts seen on MRI and SPECT-CT were opened, cleaned of all fibrotic tissue, and microfractured (*F*); spongiosa from the iliac crest was impacted into the defect (*G*); the collagen matrix was glued on top of the spongiosa graft (*H*); and the surgery was finalized with a mediolateral ligamentoplasty and a medial sliding calcaneal osteotomy. Postoperative imaging at 4 years' follow-up (*I–K*): conventional radiographs show good integration of the graft into the talus (*I*); sagittal T1 fat-suppressed MRI shows a minor residual bone marrow edema (*J*); and a sagittal DESS sequence shows a complete defect repair with an intact surface and nearly normal signal intensity (*K*).

with first-time surgery at 12 months' follow-up. The American Orthopaedic Foot and Ankle Society hindfoot score improved significantly from 63.1 points preoperatively to 86 points on follow-up. Walther and colleagues[31] reported approximately 42 cases with a minimum follow-up time of 12 months. In this cohort, the American Orthopaedic Foot and Ankle Society hindfoot score improved from 47.3 points to 88.3 points. A single report describes the use of the AMIC technique in a talar OCL revision case[32] and in a case of a rare isolated OCL of the distal tibia.[33] Other reports regarding the AMIC-aided cartilage repair technique focus on operative treatment of trochlear and retropatellar cartilage lesions of the knee joint.[34,35] Several clinical outcome studies have reported good results for short-term follow-up.[36–38] Those studies, however, addressed solely cartilaginous lesions, not combined OCLs.

The currently used operative techniques for treatment of OCLs of the talus face certain drawbacks: sacrificing healthy cartilage (osteochondral autograft transfer system and mosaicplasty), multiple-stage operative procedures (matrix-induced autologous chondrocyte transplantation and autologous chondrocyte implantation), high costs (autologous chondrocyte implantation and allograft), and limited availability (allograft). The AMIC procedure provides 2 major advantages. First, it is a 1-step procedure with no need of cartilage harvesting, potentially leading to donor site morbidity. Second, it is cost effective with no need of in vitro cell expansion.

In the described technique, cancellous bone is used to reconstruct the osseous lesion. Cancellous bone grafting for OCLs of the talus has been described elsewhere.[39,40] The rationale behind this procedure is to allow cartilage regeneration on the base of healthy bony tissue. Because cancellous bone makes a loose nonstructural graft, the authors believe that a bony reconstruction can be successfully achieved only with an adequate sealing of the graft tissue against the joint cavity, in this case with a collagen matrix. To ensure the bone graft healing properly, all fibrotic tissue from underneath the diseased cartilage needs to be removed. An open approach with an optional malleolar osteotomy may be needed to address centrally or posteriorly located large cystic lesions appropriately. An arthroscopic approach for the AMIC-technique, however, has also been described previously for the knee[41] and talus.[42]

The authors emphasize the importance for additional procedures. Most talus OCLs are posttraumatic conditions and are frequently accompanied by instability or hindfoot malalignment. Aurich and colleagues[43] regard concomitant treatment of posttraumatic deformities (malalignment), ligamentous instabilities, and the reconstruction of bony defects as compulsory. The authors share the same view. Changing a pathomechanical joint into an almost normal biomechanical joint by correcting osseous malalignment (eg, calcaneal ostetomies) and improving joint stability (lateral/medial ankle ligament reconstruction; posterior tibial tendon reconstruction) might be essential for healing of the reconstructed defect. Otherwise, remaining pathologic stress on the repair tissue could eventually lead to graft failure and new pain symptoms. Evidence for this is sparse, however. Ligament repair in cases of talus OCL accompanied by ankle joint instability has been previously described in a few cases.[44,45] Regarding corrective osteotomies, Giannini and colleagues[45] report 1 case of metatarsal osteotomy in the presence of a cavus foot.

SUMMARY

The modified AMIC technique is a promising novel method for operative treatment of OCLs of the talus. A conclusion regarding advantage over other treatment methods, however, cannot be made at this point due to lack of evidence.

REFERENCES

1. Taga I, Shino K, Inoue M, et al. Articular cartilage lesions in ankles with lateral ligament injury. An arthroscopic study. Am J Sports Med 1993;21(1):120–6 [discussion: 126–7].
2. Hintermann B, Boss A, Schafer D. Arthroscopic findings in patients with chronic ankle instability. Am J Sports Med 2002;30(3):402–9.
3. Verhagen RA, Struijs PA, Bossuyt PM, et al. Systematic review of treatment strategies for osteochondral defects of the talar dome. Foot Ankle Clin 2003;8(2): 233–42, viii–ix.
4. Flick AB, Gould N. Osteochondritis dissecans of the talus (transchondral fractures of the talus): review of the literature and new surgical approach for medial dome lesions. Foot Ankle 1985;5(4):165–85.
5. Anderson DV, Lyne ED. Osteochondritis dissecans of the talus: case report on two family members. J Pediatr Orthop 1984;4(3):356–7.
6. Woods K, Harris I. Osteochondritis dissecans of the talus in identical twins. J Bone Joint Surg Br 1995;77(2):331.
7. Abu-Shakra M, Buskila D, Shoenfeld Y. Osteonecrosis in patients with SLE. Clin Rev Allergy Immunol 2003;25(1):13–24.
8. Canale ST, Belding RH. Osteochondral lesions of the talus. J Bone Joint Surg Am 1980;62(1):97–102.
9. Hakimzadeh A, Munzinger U. 8. Osteochondrosis dissecans: results after 10 or more years. c). Osteochondrosis dissecans of the ankle joint: long-term study. Orthopade 1979;8(2):135–40 [in German].
10. Pettine KA, Morrey BF. Osteochondral fractures of the talus. A long-term follow-up. J Bone Joint Surg Br 1987;69(1):89–92.
11. Steadman JR, Rodkey WG, Rodrigo JJ. Microfracture: surgical technique and rehabilitation to treat chondral defects. Clin Orthop Relat Res 2001;(Suppl 391): S362–9.
12. Hangody L. The mosaicplasty technique for osteochondral lesions of the talus. Foot Ankle Clin 2003;8(2):259–73.
13. Hangody L, Kish G, Modis L, et al. Mosaicplasty for the treatment of osteochondritis dissecans of the talus: two to seven year results in 36 patients. Foot Ankle Int 2001;22(7):552–8.
14. Imhoff AB, Paul J, Ottinger B, et al. Osteochondral transplantation of the talus: long-term clinical and magnetic resonance imaging evaluation. Am J Sports Med 2011;39(7):1487–93.
15. Ronga M, Grassi FA. Treatment of deep cartilage defects of the ankle with matrix-induced autologous chondrocyte implantation (MACI). Foot Ankle Surg 2005;11: 29–33.
16. Giannini S, Buda R, Grigolo B, et al. Autologous chondrocyte transplantation in osteochondral lesions of the ankle joint. Foot Ankle Int 2001;22(6):513–7.
17. Raikin SM. Fresh osteochondral allografts for large-volume cystic osteochondral defects of the talus. J Bone Joint Surg Am 2009;91(12):2818–26.
18. Behrens P. Matrixgekoppelte Mikrofrakturierung. Arthroskopie 2005;18:193–7.
19. Behrens P, Bitter T, Kurz B, et al. Matrix-associated autologous chondrocyte transplantation/implantation (MACT/MACI)—5-year follow-up. Knee 2006;13(3): 194–202.
20. Gille J, Schuseil E, Wimmer J, et al. Mid-term results of Autologous Matrix-Induced Chondrogenesis for treatment of focal cartilage defects in the knee. Knee Surg Sports Traumatol Arthrosc 2010;18(11):1456–64.

21. Hepple S, Winson IG, Glew D. Osteochondral lesions of the talus: a revised classification. Foot Ankle Int 1999;20(12):789–93.
22. Saltzman CL, el-Khoury GY. The hindfoot alignment view. Foot Ankle Int 1995; 16(9):572–6.
23. Carlsson AM. Assessment of chronic pain. I. Aspects of the reliability and validity of the visual analogue scale. Pain 1983;16(1):87–101.
24. Wiewiorski M, Pagenstert G, Rasch H, et al. Pain in osteochondral lesions. Foot Ankle Spec 2011;4(2):92–9.
25. Drobnic M, Radosavljevic D, Ravnik D, et al. Comparison of four techniques for the fixation of a collagen scaffold in the human cadaveric knee. Osteoarthr Cartil 2006;14(4):337–44.
26. Knupp M, Stufkens SA, Bolliger L, et al. Classification and treatment of supramalleolar deformities. Foot Ankle Int 2011;32(11):1023–31.
27. Pagenstert G, Leumann A, Hintermann B, et al. Sports and recreation activity of varus and valgus ankle osteoarthritis before and after realignment surgery. Foot Ankle Int 2008;29(10):985–93.
28. Brostrom L. Sprained ankles. VI. Surgical treatment of "chronic" ligament ruptures. Acta Chir Scand 1966;132(5):551–65.
29. Wiewiorski M, Leumann A, Buettner O, et al. Autologous matrix-induced chondrogenesis aided reconstruction of a large focal osteochondral lesion of the talus. Arch Orthop Trauma Surg 2011;131(3):293–6.
30. Barg A, Miska M, Wiewiorski W, et al. Autologous Matrix-induced Chondrogenesis (AMIC) for Reconstruction of Osteochondral Lesions of the talus. Presented at the 18th Annual Meeting of German Society of Foot and Ankle Surgery. Dresden, Germany, March 23, 2012.
31. Walther M. Treatment option in osteochondral lesions: open ACT/AMIC. Presented at the 18th Annual Meeting of German Society of Foot and Ankle Surgery. Dresden, Germany, March 23, 2012.
32. Wiewiorski M, Miska M, Nicolas G, et al. Revision of failed osteochondral autologous transplantation procedure for chronic talus osteochondral lesion with iliac crest graft and autologous matrix-induced chondrogenesis: a case report. Foot Ankle Spec 2012;5(2):115–20.
33. Miska M, Wiewiorski M, Valderrabano V. Reconstruction of a Large Osteochondral Lesion of the Distal Tibia with an Iliac Crest Graft and Autologous Matrix-induced Chondrogenesis (AMIC): a case report. J Foot Ankle Surg 2012;51(5):680–3.
34. Benthien JP, Behrens P. Autologous Matrix-Induced Chondrogenesis (AMIC): combining microfracturing and a collagen I/III matrix for articular cartilage resurfacing. Cartilage 2010;1:65–8.
35. Benthien JP, Behrens P. Autologous matrix-induced chondrogenesis (AMIC). A one-step procedure for retropatellar articular resurfacing. Acta Orthop Belg 2010;76(2):260–3.
36. Steinwachs M, Kreuz PC. Autologous chondrocyte implantation in chondral defects of the knee with a type I/III collagen membrane: a prospective study with a 3-year follow-up. Arthroscopy 2007;23(4):381–7.
37. Niemeyer P, Pestka JM, Kreuz PC, et al. Characteristic complications after autologous chondrocyte implantation for cartilage defects of the knee joint. Am J Sports Med 2008;36(11):2091–9.
38. Gooding CR, Bartlett W, Bentley G, et al. A prospective, randomised study comparing two techniques of autologous chondrocyte implantation for osteochondral defects in the knee: periosteum covered versus type I/III collagen covered. Knee 2006;13(3):203–10.

39. Lahm A, Erggelet C, Steinwachs M, et al. Arthroscopic management of osteochondral lesions of the talus: results of drilling and usefulness of magnetic resonance imaging before and after treatment. Arthroscopy 2000;16(3): 299–304.
40. Taranow WS, Bisignani GA, Towers JD, et al. Retrograde drilling of osteochondral lesions of the medial talar dome. Foot Ankle Int 1999;20(8):474–80.
41. Piontek T, Ciemniewska-Gorzela K, Szulc A, et al. All-arthroscopic AMIC procedure for repair of cartilage defects of the knee. Knee Surg Sports Traumatol Arthrosc 2012;20(5):922–5.
42. Walther M, Becher C, Volkering C, et al. Therapie chondraler und osteochondraler Defekte am Talus durch Autologe Matrix Induzierte Chondrogenese. Fuss Sprungg 2012;10(2):121–9.
43. Aurich M, Venbrocks RA, Fuhrmann RA. Autologous chondrocyte transplantation in the ankle joint. Rational or irrational? Orthopade 2008;37(3):188, 190–5. [in German].
44. Kono M, Takao M, Naito K, et al. Retrograde drilling for osteochondral lesions of the talar dome. Am J Sports Med 2006;34(9):1450–6.
45. Giannini S, Buda R, Faldini C, et al. Surgical treatment of osteochondral lesions of the talus in young active patients. J Bone Joint Surg Am 2005;87(Suppl 2):28–41.

Index

Note: Page numbers of article titles are in **boldface** type.

A

Abrasion arthroplasty, for cystic osteochondral defects, 118
Abrasion chondroplasty, for OLTs, with debridement and microfracture, 69
ACI. See *Autologous chondrocyte implantation (ACI).*
Activity modification, for cystic osteochondral defects, 116
    for OLTs, 15
Adjunctive therapies, for articular cartilage repair, 8
    for microfracture repair, 5
Age. See *Patient age.*
Aggrecan, in articular cartilage, 2
Alignment. See *Malalignment.*
Allograft talar reconstruction, for OLTs, 100–109
        benefits of, 100
        contraindications to, 101
        cystic, 117
        indications for, 101
        limitations of, 100–101
        pitfalls of, 108
        postoperative protocol for, 107–108
        recurrent, 151–152, 155
        results of, 109
        surgical technique for, 101–108
            anterior approach for large defects, 103–108
            graft preparation options in, 101–103
Allograft transplantation, particulated juvenile articular cartilage, for OLTs, **79–87**. See also
    Particulated juvenile articular cartilage allograft transplantation (PJCAT).
Allografts, osteochondral, for cystic osteochondral defects, 118, 120
        for large, cystic, shoulder lesions, 80, 82–83
    for OLTs. See *Osteochondral autograft transfer system (OATS).*
    osteotomy of, in allograft talar reconstruction, 105, 107
    talar, for OATS, 19
        for reconstruction, 100–109. See also *Allograft talar reconstruction.*
Aluminum foil, in DeNovo graft placement, 83–84
American Orthopaedic Foot and Ankle Society (AOFAS), cyst formation and, 115
    post-ACI/MACI, 147
    post-AMIC, 155
    post-treatment, of articular cartilage injuries, 3, 6, 99, 109
AMIC. See *Autologous matrix-induced chondrogenesis (AMIC).*
Anderson classification system, of OLTs, 50–51
Angiogenesis, from shock wave therapy, for bone bruising and OCDs, 42
    for OLTs, 22
Animal models, of chondrocyte implantation, scaffold-associated, 6–7

Foot Ankle Clin N Am 18 (2013) 159–183
http://dx.doi.org/10.1016/S1083-7515(13)00011-9
1083-7515/13/$ – see front matter © 2013 Elsevier Inc. All rights reserved.

foot.theclinics.com

Moving?

Make sure your subscription moves with you!

To notify us of your new address, find your **Clinics Account Number** (located on your mailing label above your name), and contact customer service at:

Email: journalscustomerservice-usa@elsevier.com

800-654-2452 (subscribers in the U.S. & Canada)
314-447-8871 (subscribers outside of the U.S. & Canada)

Fax number: 314-447-8029

Elsevier Health Sciences Division
Subscription Customer Service
3251 Riverport Lane
Maryland Heights, MO 63043

*To ensure uninterrupted delivery of your subscription, please notify us at least 4 weeks in advance of move.

Printed and bound by CPI Group (UK) Ltd, Croydon, CR0 4YY

03/10/2024

01040436-0012